Only the Strong Survive

Ashley Biddiscombe

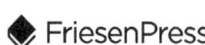
One Printers Way
Altona, MB R0G 0B0
Canada

www.friesenpress.com

Copyright © 2022 by Ashley Biddiscombe
First Edition — 2022

All rights reserved.

No part of this publication may be reproduced in any form, or by any means, electronic or mechanical, including photocopying, recording, or any information browsing, storage, or retrieval system, without permission in writing from FriesenPress.

ISBN
978-1-03-915819-1 (Hardcover)
978-1-03-915818-4 (Paperback)
978-1-03-915820-7 (eBook)

1. FAMILY & RELATIONSHIPS, ADOPTION & FOSTERING

Distributed to the trade by The Ingram Book Company

This book is dedicated to my wife, who I could not do this life without.

INTRODUCTION

Are you looking for a story about two people who fall in love, find joy, and live the fairy tale life? Then put this book down now.

I've always been one for raw honesty. This is a story about the forks in the road, and how I realized I was meant for something different than I set out for myself. It's about how relationships grow and change, and how you must fight for love, and how we go into parenting naïve, not fully understanding how hard it can be. This is a story about never giving up.

It's Saturday morning, and I'm sitting at the dining room table with a cold waffle and a cold coffee. Isn't that the parenting norm? I've tried to start this paragraph eight times already, but a tiny boy with pink hair—*yep, I said pink*—keeps asking me for "more drink," and a sassy girl is telling me she can pour her own cereal—the crunch under my feet on the kitchen floor is telling me she's missed the bowl. There is a teenager asleep in the basement, and my other half is at work this morning. Our house wasn't always this full, this noisy, or this messy, but here we are.

We all grow up dreaming about what it will be like when we are adults. We create a magical world, and the perfect fairy tale. You grow up, you get married, you get pregnant with your happy little bump. The kids grow up and go away to college, you retire, and live out your years . . . . But what happens when your story is different? You grow up, you get married, you can't get pregnant,

Ashley Biddiscombe

you turn to adoption, and your children's special needs will likely keep you all under the same roof forever? No one prepares you for that fairy tale.

Let me take you on a journey of two girls who fell in love, struggled with infertility, dove into adoption, and are now riding the rollercoaster of special needs parenting.

This book is for those who have seen the ugly face of infertility and survived its heartbreak. It's for those who have jumped on the adoption train, and have opened their homes to trauma, open adoption, transitions, and a lot of paperwork—and for those special needs parents fighting every day for inclusion, advocating for a better life, and in the trenches of the "the hard."

Get cozy with your morning coffee, or evening wine, or your morning tequila sunrise—there's no judgment here—and I'll take you along for the winding tale of our story.

My hope is that no matter where you are in your own journey, you feel a little less alone in yours knowing someone else in the world has a story like yours. Someone who has been in the depths, unsure if they would get out, and has been on a not-so-typical path, raising not-so-typical kids.

ONE:
Blue Skies and Full of Hope

Where else do we start but the beginning?

It was the early 2000s, the brink of cellphones and the Internet. Ashley and I met in high school, and I was fascinated from the moment I saw her. She was different than the other friends that I had grown up with, and I couldn't explain it. Looking back, I had a massive crush on her, but being gay and open about it wasn't an option—especially at that age, and according to social norms. Ellen DeGeneres had only come out a few years prior, it was still all over the tabloids about how her career had taken a plunge for wanting to live her truth as a gay woman. There was only one openly gay girl in our high school. It was taboo, and almost like wearing the scarlet letter. So, you just tried to fit into the straight life that everyone expected you to be a part of. We grew closer as we navigated the woes of high school, but after graduation, it was clear there was something more. We hid our relationship, we fought about our relationship, and we tried to figure out how not to be together. None of it worked for us—we just wanted each other.

We drove around in Ashley's old Sunbird. She had worked hard on it all throughout high school. The body work took forever, and it was known as the "primer mobile" until she was finally able to afford to get it painted. She suffered through my riding lessons and horse shows on weekends just so we could hang out together. When I bought my first condo, we went out and got my first Christmas tree. We threw it over the balcony to get it inside, and broke the top off. We taped it back on. It wasn't straight, but it held the star. We travelled around for months, searching any humane society and pet shop within a two-hour radius for the Tuxedo kitten Ashley wanted, only to find him ten minutes from home. Ashley named him James, like James Bond. He had a bowtie and drank his water out of a martini glass. He went everywhere with us. James was followed by my tabby cat, Kisha. Ashley got Felix, and I found Tequila soon after. Our condos were down the hall from each other, and we would travel back and forth, shaking a cat treat bag, with all four cats in tow. Our first Valentine's Day, Ashley filled my condo with candles and made a picnic on the floor with Swiss Chalet before coming to get me at work. I still don't know how she didn't burn the place down.

When we finally decided to come out, we were scared. We had been convinced we had been keeping it all under wraps, but when we told our closest friends, they laughed and responded, "Yeah, we know, it's about time." We were in our early twenties. We drove around with our windows down and music loud. We lived off microwave dinners and brunches with hangovers. We were working to live, had no responsibilities and all the time in the world.

In 2009, Ashley proposed under the starry sky at the end of the dock on my favourite lake. Same-sex marriages were still relatively new—especially when you weren't from a huge, flashy city. We would go to wedding shows, and you had to ask vendors if they did gay weddings. Some would say no, and you would just have to accept that and move onto the next. Picking vendors involved with our wedding had to be done with care. Our teamwork skills were impeccable, really—but that's what you get when two women plan their wedding.

Only the Strong Survive

We got asked regularly, "Who is going to wear the dress?" We shook are heads and smiled. "We both are." People had no idea what to expect at a lesbian wedding, which gave us all the freedom to do whatever we wanted without being tied down to tradition. But questions like that make me realize how far we've come since then.

In 2010, on the perfect October day, the skies were that perfect shade of blue—not a cloud in the sky. We were having our perfect day. We walked down the aisle to Bruno Mars's "Just the Way You Are." We took pictures under the fall colours, ate the best cake I've ever tasted, and danced the night away. At twenty-six, we were starting our marriage off with a bang—a day that people have talked about years after the party was done and the guests had stumbled home.

We woke up the next morning still groggy from the night before. Who knew weddings could be so exhausting? It would be a lie if I didn't say we may have thrown all the gifted money around like we had won the lottery. Instead of a honeymoon, we started renovations on our recently-bought house—all the motivated things people in their twenties do. We ended the days relaxing with our friends who lived down the street, who had also just gotten married. We sat on couches in our empty, torn-up living room with a TV tray and our leftover wedding cake as we passed around a champagne bottle, laughing and talking about the future. Kind of sounds like a romantic comedy, doesn't it?

We were newlyweds, had jobs we loved, fur kids, and endless energy. We fostered kittens for a local rescue. We went cottaging at the beach with our friends, drank too much at nightclubs, and took sign language classes for fun. Your twenties have this magic to them that you don't fully see until they are gone. You are trying to figure out who you are, but still have a lifetime to figure it all out. We didn't realize how good we had it back then. If someone were to ask me "if you could go back in time for a vacation, where would you go? Early twenties, hands-down—pass me the Smirnoff, I'll be at the beach.

I was working two jobs. One was to pay the bills and the other was purely passion—as a therapeutic horseback riding instructor at a local charity. I instructed children and adults with disabilities of all kinds. The job found me by accident when I was twenty, and saw me into my thirties. It was the kind of job that I knew I was meant for. I don't brag about too many things, but that job . . . I was good at it, and I loved it with every fibre of my being.

Having the ability to watch small miracles happen each lesson is a privilege that many don't get to witness. Over the years, I have watched unspoken bonds between horse and rider that cannot be explained. I have watched a mother be able to hug her child for the first time without his body convulsing, with tears of happiness falling to her cheeks. I've witnessed a four-year-old boy saying his first word to his pony, and celebrate in the joy with his parents. I have watched a girl get lifted from her wheelchair and take her first steps on a horse, and the sense of freedom that provides. I've watched a girl with visual impairment put full faith into a thousand-pound animal to be her eyes, and full faith in me to keep her safe.

Without knowing it at the time, the parents who walked through those doors—the ones I admired for their strength—would be the same parents I would be sitting in waiting rooms with years later. But what I know now is that it wasn't miracles I was witnessing. It was years of blood, sweat, tears, and advocating that I was seeing finally come to fruition—and those parent tears were so much deeper than the feeling of joy. If I could go back knowing what I know now, I would have hugged those parents harder, I would have celebrated bigger, and taken in those moments differently. Every step in life has a purpose.

When we weren't working and home, we were with our families. We would fly out west for long weekends to spend time with our niece and nephew as much as we could. At family gatherings, I would sit with Ashley's cousins and their babies and love every minute of it. On my side, I was the oldest cousin, with almost two decades between me and the youngest. We were always surrounded by kids. Ashley was ready to start a family. I was still enjoying my twenties to the fullest. I knew I wanted kids, but was I really ready to commit to that right now? I still didn't feel like an adult—but I did at the same time. Your twenties can be a weird time.

In April 2011, we found ourselves in the waiting room of a fertility clinic, the odd baby pictures scattered on the pale pink walls. We got paperwork to fill out from the receptionist, who smiled kindly at us before we nervously sat down. This clinic was a forty-five-minute drive away—the closest one at the time. There were very few fertility clinics in our area, and travelling was part of the deal.

We sat and waited for the doctor. I scanned the room, which had the odd couple or woman on her own waiting. The doctor called us back to his office for our first consultation. We talked about our hopes to conceive, and listened to the process and testing we were going to have to do to get started. Bloodwork and ultrasounds seemed simple enough. We talked about using donor sperm and got more information on the cryobanks and storage at the clinic. He talked about percentages and success rate with confidence, ultimately making us feel confident as well. We left a little wary about if we were ready, but confident it was going to work. We would start this journey and we would become parents. We were young, healthy, and full of hope.

We decided I would be the one to carry. Ashley had never really wanted to be pregnant—and I did, wholeheartedly. I completed the testing required, which all looked good, and then moved onto calling the cryobank. It's a funny process, shopping for sperm. There are many ways you can narrow down your profiles—by race, eye colour, hair colour, job, interests. We decided on taking our pictures, and had them find donors who had similar facial profiles as we did. Regardless of who carried the child, the donor's features were close to both of us, making it feel a little more personal. We got sent a page of donor numbers, and we clicked on each one opening to see a picture, complete with general information about the donor and their medical history. It was like reading his stats—as if we were picking players for a sports team. We narrowed it down to donor 9923—he was our guy, the one who was going to help us make a family. He had had successful births already. It had to happen. We paid a whopping nine hundred dollars per vial—we bought in bulk, just in case it didn't happen right away, and it was shipped to the clinic so it was ready for us.

When it was time for our first monitored cycle, we set our alarms for 5 a.m. If we were going to get to the clinic and back before work, we had to be on the road for 5:30 a.m. each day—forty-five minutes there and back. We agreed that the drive in the winter would be impossible—so late spring, summer, and early fall would be our limit for travel. *But it wouldn't take that long, would it?*

Our alarms went off and we were on our way. We were up before the sun and needed coffee before we hit the highway. We stopped for coffee and breakfast sandwiches. There is something eerily quiet about the roads at that time of the morning—most of the city is still asleep, and only the commuters or shift workers are travelling. The drive to London from our city wasn't invigorating by any means—highway, farms, more highway. As we drove, the sun rose behind us, creating a glow of pinks and oranges. It was always my favourite part of the drive.

We rolled into the parking lot and went through the back door to head into the clinic to the waiting room. The receptionist greeted us and waited for the nurse to call us back. The waiting room had a few other women sitting, looking at their phones. At this time in the morning, we were all there for the same thing . . . bloodwork and internal ultrasounds. The nurse called my name and motioned for Ash to come back with us. She was going to be allowed in every room with me. We were doing this together, and she was going to be a part of the process, start to finish. The nurse ushered us into a tiny room big enough for two chairs and bloodwork supplies. She chatted happily as she put the rubber band on my arm for the blood draw. *Well, that wasn't too bad.*

"We will rotate arms each day. Don't pick up anything heavy—especially later in the week—or you will pop a vein, and those bruises are pretty nasty. You'll like long sleeves during cycle. You tend to look like you have track marks." She smiled. This staff was sure happy in the mornings.

She led us down a narrow hallway. It was brightly lit from the big windows—you could see the last of the sunrise. It created a glow on the floor. We passed a couple of small rooms and along the hallway there were painted baby hands with names and dates along the walls. It was all the successful families who had come back to say hi. She sat us down in another small waiting area that had padded benches instead of chairs, tucked away in a little nook. There were two ultrasound rooms in front of us. The ultrasound technician would call someone back into the room and then head into the other to do an ultrasound. She rotated between the two rooms with ease. When she called us back, she explained where to put my clothes from the waist down, climb up onto the bed, and pointed at the paper I could use to cover myself with. There is nothing that feels less secure than a paper blanket. The room was dimly lit, but it was cozy. The bed faced a deep purple wall with a large-screen TV on it. The far corner, where I was going to put my clothes, had a curtain I could close for privacy, and there was an extra chair beside the bed, where Ashley could sit. She wasn't gone too long before popping back in. She flicked on the screen, and you could see a mirror image from her tiny screen up on the wall. She started the internal ultrasound and grey images moved around the screen. Then a round circle, with other small circles inside, appeared. "There is the right ovary. You've got some small follicles." You could see a yellow line drag and stop, drag and stop—and then she would freeze the screen. "I'm measuring the follicles so we can keep track of their size every day, to see how many are growing before ovulation." That made sense, as she moved onto the left side. Easy enough—we would just watch and see what happened throughout the week. Day after day, we would make the drive, do bloodwork, and head to ultrasound. By day seven, I still wasn't having too much success with my follicles growing to optimal sizes, and at the end of the cycle, we were back in the doctor's office.

"We are going to start you on Clomid. It's a simple pill you take every day, and it will help those eggs grow." The doctor was pretty matter-of-fact. He handed us a prescription, and we were on our way. This cycle was done, but I would call them on day three of my period, and we would have our next plan to come back in for our first official round.

My cycle was not regular, and I was not patient. It took about two months before we were heading back to London. Just as we had done before, we were up with the sun, coffees and breakfast in hand, and headed down the highway. The first round wasn't too bad, but being poked and prodded at 6 a.m. everyday wasn't easy. Even though you alternated your arms for bloodwork, they were tender by the end of the cycle—even the cotton ball and tape hurt by day seven. All it took was one busted up vein for your arms to be purple. And does that stop them from poking you again? No. But you sit there and smile and then say thank you, like they are giving you a gift every morning.

You learn very quickly which nurses are good at blood draws. The nursing staff was made of up a few women and one man. I am sure the men that come through the fertility clinic appreciated having a male nurse to talk to. However, he was the absolute worst at bloodwork. Brad was always so chatty and upbeat in the morning—but *man*, did he have an angle wrong or something, which made his blood draws twice as painful as anyone else in the clinic. When I would be sitting in the waiting room, seeing the rotating nurses calling people back, I would sit praying I got someone else—and when I didn't, I cringed. I don't know how the words "God damnit Brad, find the vein, Brad, fucking hell, Brad . . ." didn't leave my lips on a regular basis. He quickly gained the nickname "Stabby Bradley" on our drives home.

During the first cycle, we had an egg; it was big and ready. Ideally, we wanted a measurement between sixteen and eighteen—and we were there, and it was time for our first IUI. An IUI is short for inter-uterine insemination. They basically take a tube and push it past your cervix to get the goods right up in there. It is as uncomfortable as it sounds. On the day of the IUI, we were moved to a room we hadn't been in before—Ashley beside me, and one of my favourite nurses by our side.

Afterward, you are told to lay there for fifteen minutes before leaving. So, you lay there trying to act casual, looking up at the ceiling until the timer goes off. We were excited. *This could be it, this could be our baby.*

After the excitement of the IUI, they send you home—and all you do is wait. It's out of everyone's hand now. After two weeks, you head back for a pregnancy test, and then you wait again—impatiently, I might add—for the results. Then you get *the* phone call.

"Hi, Ashley, just calling you with your results. I'm sorry—it's negative this time."

You thank them and tell them you will see them in the next round. The first time you get the call, you feel disappointed—but the first cycle wasn't too bad. *We could definitely do it all over again.* We were still plenty hopeful.

The months ticked on, and we watched spring turn to summer, then to fall. The sunrise changed with the seasons, and our fall drives were in the dark on the way to the clinic, and the sun would rise on the way home. Cycle after cycle, needle after needle, the phone calls were always the same: "I'm sorry, it's negative." Every time, I'd hang up the phone and take a deep breath in, letting it out with a few tears. I was starting to feel defeated. I was young, I was healthy—*why wasn't this working*? We were setting up the perfect cycle, and every time, it failed.

Our last cycle before we decided to take the winter off was a long one. I don't know if my body was just used to the dose of Clomid or *what* was going on, but seven days in, there was still no change—my eggs refused to grow. They wanted to go for a few more days, just in case my hormones were all just delayed. Not every cycle is the same. During this round, I had blown a vein at work lifting a rider onto a horse, and the bruise went from my elbow all the way up my bicep. Most of my bruising was only tender—but that one was painful. Even putting my arms into the sleeves of my shirt hurt.

"We've got to let that arm heal. We're going to use your right arm only going forward." I cringed as the nurse took my blood yet again. By this point, it didn't matter who did the blood draw—they all hurt like hell. "I can move to your foot if you want." *My foot? Oh, fuck that—come on, right arm, you can take this.*

Finally, day ten, we called our defeat—not one follicle grew, and an IUI wouldn't be happening. We decided to take the winter off, regroup—and in the spring, we would try again with higher drug dosages. I would have a love-hate relationship with these breaks. Every time we weren't trying, we were missing an opportunity—and it started to become an obsession. They don't tell you about how the drive to keep going changes you. With every no, you become more desperate for a yes. You lay on the ultrasound bed, and you watch your eggs on the screen growing each day. *Will that be the one that finally makes us parents?* The doctors add more drugs to your cycle, and you take them if it means you will finally get the *yes*. With every drug comes a new side effect—water retention, weight gain, acne, clearer skin, hot flashes. Hot flashes were the worst. It was always at night, and would feel like a furnace deep in my core. Starting slow at first, then my whole body would be on fire—and off the sheets would come, drenched in sweat, only for them to pass just as fast. It would happen on and off all night long. No one is less fun than a woman jacked up on hormones who isn't sleeping.

When we moved on to injectable medication, I could not hype myself up to be able to inject myself with the needles. Ashley tried a couple of times, but felt horrible about hurting me. I often called up our friend Jill, who is a nurse, and she would come over, give me my needle in under a second, hang out for a bit, and be on her way. True best friends will stab you with needles on your baby journey.

We started back up in the spring with the same long, boring drive. By this point, we could've done it with our eyes closed. I'll be honest—we even counted roadkill to keep ourselves busy. I had every farm and every bend in the road memorized. More needles, more drugs, and more ultrasounds, followed by more *no* phone calls. I had started buying pregnancy tests and hiding them in the bathroom, just so that I could know before the phone call came in. That way, I could process, have a cry, and be able to move on with my day.

The further we got into our journey, the harder I was finding it to be happy for our friends who were getting pregnant so easily. I could feel the jealousy rise. *How could it be so easy for them? What do you mean it was an accident?* We were spending thousands of dollars. We were putting in all the effort we possibly could and getting nowhere. I couldn't look at baby pictures and "we are expecting" announcements without feeling angry. When would it be our turn?

We had people with good intentions, not understanding our heartbreak, trying to give us words of encouragement. "It'll happen." "You guys deserve this." And then the not-so-helpful comments. "Oh, that sounds hard. Man, I would get pregnant if we just passed each other in the hall."

Three and a half years, many useless cycles, and nine unsuccessful IUIs later, we decided to switch clinics. Maybe there was something we were missing—maybe a different doctor could help us. Our pregnancy journey was looking a lot less shiny with excitement, and a lot more like pain and heartbreak mixed with desperation. I didn't want to leave the clinic we were at, but we just felt stuck. Saying goodbye to the staff was harder than I expected. They had been through so many ups and downs with us. We would bring them coffees in the early mornings. They always greeted us with smiling faces and chitchat. They were full of compassion, and I trusted them. I would even miss Stabby Bradley. Having to start all over felt overwhelming. We didn't know what we needed, but we needed more.

TWO:
Only the Strong Survive

It took four months to get into the new fertility clinic closer to home. The drive was much shorter, and we didn't have to worry about the winter weather anymore. The building wasn't new and bright like the old one. It was older, and the outside was a chocolate shade of brown that reminded me of panelling from the 1980s. The inside was the same outdated colours, and it was well-worn and in desperate need of an update. The waiting room had beige textured wallpaper and a faded painting of a cottage hung on the wall. There were no windows, and the dim lights create dark corners in the room. The receptionist was in a tiny plexiglass box in the corner, and she would keep the window closed unless she was helping someone. There were no smiles, no happy hellos. The new doctor was not as friendly, either—she was direct, kind of socially awkward. She didn't look us in the eye while we talked, and spoke in a direct, to-the-point way. Knowing what I know now, I think she may have been autistic. She was the best in the area—and was there to be my doctor, not my friend.

She scanned through our file and ordered more testing to be done before she would consider trying a cycle. There had to be a reason we weren't getting pregnant. She ordered a biopsy to make sure I didn't have a hostile uterus.

"We will go up like an IUI and take a tiny bit of tissue to have it analyzed. Take two Tylenol and two Advil beforehand. It is uncomfortable, but not too bad," she explained. I really should have questioned that procedure more, but I had been through so much already, I just nodded in agreement.

On the day of the biopsy, I took my painkillers as instructed and stripped down naked from the waist down, as I had for the last three years. Everyone else had been up there so far, one more nurse wasn't going to make a difference. I laid the scratchy paper square around my legs and waited. There's nothing like a freezing-cold doctor's office to really get you ready. The nurse came in, making small talk. She knew what this was all about. Looking back, I'm glad I didn't. I will save you the gory details of what happened next, but I will tell you I have never been closer to kicking someone in the face before—and there's a reason they sugar coat things. I have often wondered if the doctors ordering these procedures have ever had to endure them themselves. Do they actually know what "not too bad" feels like?

The clinic called me a couple of days later. I was cleared of anything that could hinder our chances of carrying to full term. The had doctor decided to change my medications to try a different cocktail, and we were ready to start what we didn't realize would be our last cycle.

On the first day, Ash drove me in like she did at every other appointment. It would be the opposite at this clinic—ultrasound first, then bloodwork. And they were on two separate floors of the building. We walked into the waiting room where the ultrasounds took place. It had one tiny window in the far end that didn't really let any natural light in. The walls were painted a dull sunshine yellow that needed to be freshened up. Between the old paint, brown carpet, and fluorescent lighting, it was less than visually appealing. It was much bigger than the other clinic, and had multiple rooms and ultrasound technicians. When they called my name to go back, Ashley stood up to come back with me and the nurse shook her head. I had to go alone. Ashley nodded at me reassuringly.

"It's OK. I will wait here." I felt like our team was getting split up, and I didn't like it.

I was led to a small, box-like changeroom with curtain. "Change in here into the gown. You can leave your stuff in here and then go to room two" The nurse pointed in the direction and disappeared. I changed and headed to room two. The technician was already inside, waiting. There were no warm purple walls, and no big screens or warm salt lamps. There was a bed and a machine. I got up on the bed, and we started the ultrasound. This technician was a little rougher than I was used to as she moved the wand around. I turned my head to see if I could see the screen. It was titled away.

"Can you see anything?" I heard the clicking and freezeframe tap as she measured.

"I can't tell you. You will have to wait for the phone call later." All I could think was *I don't like this*. We finished, and I went back to change and meet Ashley so we could head downstairs. Again, she waited in the waiting room while I got my blood drawn in a little cubicle. The nurse was nice, but I suddenly missed the nurses in London. This all felt too foreign. I knew it was going to be different, but I wasn't expecting it to be so clinical and cold. We headed back to the Jeep, feeling wildly out of place and uneasy.

"I mean, I can still come and just wait in the waiting room?" She looked at me supportively as I shook my head.

"That's silly. You should just go into work. I mean we've done this part before, and we don't even know about any changes until they call me with updates later in the day, since they don't tell you anything in the ultrasound room." It made sense, and we agreed I would be on my own for everything, and would only relay the information back to her. It no longer felt like a journey we would be doing together, but a scary one in a new clinic, with new nurses, on my own . . . and I didn't really have an option to say otherwise.

Things happened fast—too fast. The medication cocktail that they came up with had put my ovaries into overdrive. Everything felt full and heavy by day seven. I couldn't even bend over without feeling like there were huge tennis balls inside me. The ultrasound technician looked at me with a concerned expression. "You must be uncomfortable. Your ovaries are the size of oranges. I'm counting twenty-six eggs." *Wait . . . what? Twenty-six?! What happens with that many?* She sent the results up to the doctor right away, and I got a phone call shortly after.

"This doesn't happen often, but your body has reacted too well to these drugs. It would be irresponsible to move forward with IUI as a possibility, but we can do an unscheduled IVF. You need to make this decision by later today, or we will miss our chance. It will cost half the price. I will get nurse to email you the prices. We need an answer as soon as possible to make arrangements."

Invitro fertilization was never on my list of things I was willing to pursue. It seemed too invasive, too expensive, and too out of reach. But now it was in reach, it wasn't too expensive. But was I willing to do it? I had to wait to talk to Ashley. I couldn't make this choice on my own. This was our choice together. I sat down, shifting, trying to get comfortable on our bed. I just needed these follicles out of my body. I explained what had happened, and we weighed the pros and cons and talked about how if we were going to do something extreme, *this* was the time. We decided it was the time and I picked up the phone and made the call. We were instantly scheduled in for the next night, February 11, 2014, at eight o'clock at night. And what I didn't realize is this appointment would change the course of my life forever.

The next day, while I waited nervously, I made the mistake of googling the procedure. I am the kind of person who needs to know what is coming. I'd rather know what it all looks like, good

Only the Strong Survive

and bad. I even need to know how a book ends when I start it. My wife calls me an "ending ruiner." I say I hate surprises. I did my best to wrap my head around what was going to happen—but as the time ticked on, the reality of our decision kicked in, and I felt the jitters set in. We were told to bring a blanket with us for my comfort and extra warmth. I picked a new, soft, beige one I had just bought. It was the perfect lap size. I put comfortable clothes on, and off we went into the February cold.

When we arrived, they had me sit in a recliner-type chair as they put in my IV, and they prepped the procedure room. What happened next my wife cannot talk about to this day. It is a trauma trigger for her, and I respect that. I talk about it because it's the only way I can process my grief—otherwise, it would be locked in box high on a top shelf never to be opened again.

They had me lay down on the bed. Ashley was on my left side, in a chair ,so she could be there with me. The nurse in charge of my IV meds was on my right. The door to the embryo room on my right-hand side was open, and there were two technicians inside, waiting. At my feet, the doctor and two nurses. It was a full house. The doctors told me that they were going to give drugs so I would barely remember a thing afterwards—kind of like a roofie, I assumed. Funny how you believe that's how it works.

For those who have never experienced IVF, let me fill you in on how it's done. The doctor takes a twelve-inch extraction needle, and it's inserted through the vaginal wall and into the ovary to extract each egg. It is then put into a Petrie dish and mixed with sperm, and then you wait to see which eggs fertilize and grow. The days following, they either do an IUI to implant or freeze your embryos for future implantation. I'm sure there are a lot more technical ways to explain it, but let's keep it simple.

As I lay there, I remember thinking *OK, just breathe through this—childbirth will be so much harder. This is nothing. You've got this . . . . End goal, baby.* The doctor inserted the needle for the first time, and I can tell you I felt it. This side had six eggs to extract, which meant the needle was taken out and put in six times. Halfway through the right ovary, I looked up at the nurse at my head, watching my IV, and begged for more medication. She said I was tapped out of pain meds and couldn't have anymore. She looked down at me with the look of *I'm sorry* in her eyes. It was just me and my ability to bear it. My body began to shake from the pain, but I stayed quiet. I had to stay still, considering there was a twelve-inch needle inside of me.

"First side is done," the doctor announced. *What the fuck?! I can't do this; I can't take the pain. Stay still don't move. You can do this. Breathe.* As they moved onto the left ovary, tears ran down my face as I looked up at the panelled ceiling, my poor wife in the corner watching and helpless. *Why aren't the drugs working? I can remember all of this. I'm not groggy or anything . . . . So much pain.* Don't ask me how long it took to finish the procedure. It felt like eternity.

"We are done. We have eleven eggs. You did amazing. I have never seen someone get it through it like that. Women normally scream." *Did she really just say that?*

"We are just going to finish up, and we will get you to walk to the bathroom with the nurse, then to the recovery chair." *You are going to make me walk? Like, on my feet, all the way to the bathroom, after that?*

And with that, I was propped to a sitting position and helped off the table by a nurse who then led me to the bathroom to clean myself up. We won't talk about the amount of blood I left behind, as my poor wife, who was white as a sheet made her way to the recovery chairs, trying so extremely hard to be the strong one. I eventually made it to the chair, and we sat in horrified silence with my beige fluffy blanket as the nurse removed my IV and we waited for the OK to go home.

Only the Strong Survive

The days that followed were horrendous. My whole body swelled up, and I didn't recognize myself in the mirror. I felt like a warrior. Battled and bruised, but a little lost and empty. I'm sure it was a trauma response, looking back. I took a couple days off work, then headed back, pretending like I was OK as we waited to find out about our embryos. Eleven eggs—those were rather good odds. *We should be able to get a few embryos with that. I will never have to do this again. We can freeze the rest.*

Day one: "Hi Ashley, it's the embryo clinic. I just wanted to give you the update. You officially have four fertilized eggs. We will keep monitoring their progress, and I will call you tomorrow." Four eggs meant four possible babies. Less than what I would have expected—but four was a solid number.

Day two: "Good morning, Ashley—just wanted to let you know one of your embryos stopped progressing. You have three doing well—once we get to day five, we will freeze, and we will wait until your next cycle, to give your body a break." *OK, come on, guys. We just have to make it a few more days.*

Day three: "Hi Ashley, you've got two strong embryos. You lost the third" . . . *Shit, OK, two. That's still two chances.*

Day four: "Hello . . . I'm sorry to have to tell you this, but all of your embryos are gone."

I sat at my desk at work, staring at my phone. My body went numb, and I had the instant feeling that I had to get out of there. I stumbled down the hall to my boss's office.

"Are you OK if I step out for a bit?" The words fumbled out of my mouth. When you work in a small office, your coworkers become more of an extension of your family. My boss looked at me, knowing something wasn't right.

"What's wrong? are you OK?" She rose to stand.

I remember saying, "My embryos are gone. I can't have a baby," and she scooped me into her arms, and I sobbed—the kind of cry that make your whole body heave. She firmly instructed me to go to my parents' house, since Ashley wasn't home yet—and, like all good boss moms do, she insisted she would take care of the rest. There was no way she was going to let me stay at work.

Ashley found me later that night curled into the fetal position on our bed. At this point, I couldn't hold back the ugly crying anymore, and it had overtaken in me. I had never felt so defeated in my entire life. Like every ounce of me had shattered, and I was left empty. I knew in that moment I was done. We had poured thirty-five thousand dollars into treatments. My body was wrecked, and parts of me were so jaded, it would take years to recover mentally and emotionally—some of the mental scars never fully going away. I was left with a beige fluffy blanket with a blood stain I couldn't seem to get out, no matter how hard I tried. I could've gotten rid of the blanket—but I still can't seem to do that, either.

Two weeks later, we sat across from the doctor in her office. She wanted to go over everything. No part of me wanted to be there. I was numb as she opened our file.

"This wasn't an optimal cycle. Normally, we give more drugs to improve the quality of your eggs. We can do the same medication cocktail now that we know it works for you, but alter the amounts and try again with a standard IUI." *Wait—so you knew it wasn't an "optimal" cycle, but you offered to do IVF anyway, knowing it would most likely fail?* I stared at her blankly. I could feel myself bubble with frustration. I was so beyond done with the process, I couldn't even hide it.

"I'm done. I don't want to do this anymore." It came out of me in an angry, flat tone, and all I wanted to do was get out of that office. She shifted, looking at me, baffled.

"But you had results—we can just . . ." *Did she have any regard of what she just put me through? What my body just went through?*

"I'm done." I didn't hear the rest of what she had to say because I had stopped listening. I was done with needles, medications, the ultrasounds, the "I'm sorry" phone calls. I didn't want to be touched and looked at with sympathy. I didn't want to sit in waiting rooms, and for my body to not feel like my own. We left the office and drove silently home.

A couple years later, I sat down in a tattoo parlour chair and handed over my forearm. Something in me was saying, *if you can survive four years of infertility torture, you need a scar to prove you can do anything.* I think I had the drive to claim my body back as my own. This was my choice—my words,—and I was doing it in my time. The tattoo artist laid out the stencil and started. He asked me if I was OK. I smiled. *I've dealt with my bigger needles than this*, I thought, but only nodded. Ten minutes later, my forearm read, *Only the Strong Survive.* A reminder that I can get through anything. After all . . . I was one of the few that didn't scream.

THREE:
Where Do We Go from Here?

The months that followed my epic fall from grace were far from pretty. It was harder to slap that grin-and-bear it smile on than it had been in the past. Even though it was my choice to stop, depression consumed me—and coming down from all the hormones didn't help. Ashley and I both retreated into our own grief. This wasn't something I could express, nor something I wanted to talk about. I needed to sit in it. She didn't know how to help me, and I didn't want her to. I knew she felt a deep guilt about all we had been through, but I never blamed her once. It was always my body, and my final choice. I wasn't grieving not being able to have a biological child. I grieved not being able to be pregnant. I knew with every fibre of my being that even with the possibility of trying another cycle, my body was telling me *no*, this was not going to happen. Being pregnant would never be in the cards for me, and it was time to move through the motions to try to accept that.

When I was little and playing Barbies, it was always the same. Barbie would fall in love and would have the perfect wedding, followed by balled-up clothes stuffed under her dress, making a big round belly. I would look at biology books and see the stages of pregnancy and the growing fetus. I wanted to know what it felt like to feel the baby kick. The idea of childbirth never scared me. But now, the dream that I had had for so long was out of reach, and I wasn't sure how to process that. Almost four years, we had had a plan, and we had stuck to it—and now what? We no longer had morning drives together, we were no longer working towards a common goal, and we no longer felt on the same page. It was like looking into the dark hole of the abyss without having any clue what we were looking for.

As a couple, we felt alone. We didn't really have many same-sex couples we knew who were going down the same route as we were, and we didn't have any straight friends who were having fertility issues, either. They supported us the best way that they could. People in your life always want to give you words of hope—the "it'll get better" speech. I just needed someone to come sit in the hole of grief with me and let me vent and have a good cry. I think I said, "Fuck you, you don't know" in my head more times than I should admit—even to the people I love the most. At the end of the day, they didn't know our full story, and I couldn't find the words to share it. All I could do was pull away. I was broken. My body couldn't do the one thing we should be able to achieve as human beings.

So many people had touched my body over the years that it no longer felt like my own. Human contact was just too much. Even with a hug, I could feel myself recoil and my entire being reject it. I didn't want to be touched. There were days grief and depression felt like I was five thousand feet below the ocean, struggling to get to the surface and struggling to breathe. Other times, it felt like I was staring into the void of nothingness, but had no desire to leave. If someone had said, "Go put yourself in bed for a month, and we will come get you later," I would've dropped everything and put the covers over my head and not come out. Instead, I pulled myself out of bed every morning and pretended like I was OK.

Ashley Biddiscombe

It was only a couple of weeks after our IVF fail that I was supposed to be going to my cousin's baby shower. We had grown up extremely close—like, best-friend close. I had kept her in the loop over the years about our baby journey, and she was always quick to lend an ear. I picked up the phone and called her, telling her what had happened, and that I couldn't make the trip. I was happy for her, but I just couldn't do it. She was sad but understanding. I was relieved, but once I hung up, my phone started going off continuously from other family members, telling me that I was going to let her down if I wasn't there. I knew everyone knew what we had just gone through, but no one understood the magnitude of how my life had just changed. Nobody seemed to understand why I couldn't just show up to the baby shower, and how I could be so selfish by not supporting her. For the first time in our journey, I was standing up for my own wellbeing and my own mental health, and it felt like no one was listening.

The thought of even being around newborn onesies, blankets, bottles, and everyone celebrating made my whole being ache unbearably. There was no way I could be there and survive. I felt like I would literally break into a thousand pieces—and that wasn't fair to my cousin, who was so happy and so excited. I held strong and didn't go, and I know to this day I had made the right choice.

We tried to move on, and we poured ourselves back into life the best we could. We put away the odd baby item we had bought, tucked away out of sight. We took our young niece for overnight visits and played the awesome aunt role well. The pull to have one of our own wasn't going away. I wanted a family of our own. I wanted our house to feel full of laughter and the sound little feet padding down the hallway. I wanted snuggles on the couch and bedtime baths. I wanted to go to parks and swimming lessons. I wanted to watch my wife with our children as I watched her with everyone else's.

One afternoon, we were in the hot tub. The snow was still on the ground, and the air was cold, but the sun and water were warm. I looked at Ashley. "What about adoption?"

Now, I'm going to stop here for a moment to take a small detour, and make it very clear for those in the back. Infertility and adoption are two different journeys . . . one does not replace the other. You can be happy and love your family and life, and still struggle with your infertility.

Women who have had one biological child can still struggle with their infertility, whether they want more children or not.

Women who choose to not have any children can still struggle with their infertility.

Grief is not linear, and you cannot turn it on and off. It has peaks and valleys—sometimes, it feels like chasms and mountains. I can feel like full-on fire, and other times, a dull ache that you barely notice.

Infertility does not define my life, but it's still relevant even today, and I can't say if it will be forever or not. I can do almost anything I set my mind to—hell, I chose to write this book. I can be almost anyone for myself, and for other people. I can be Super Woman, and on other days, struggle to do the easiest of tasks. It doesn't mean there aren't a few dark places I choose not to go to for myself. Infertility did not stop me from rescuing horses . . . cats . . . people . . . it didn't stop me from producing art and filling galleries. It doesn't stop me from loving family and friends and their kids. It did, however, teach me my own threshold, and to stand up for my own needs, so I don't fall down a rabbit hole. I did that for a year and then some. It's pretty dark down there. Zero stars—not recommended.

In the last twelve years since our infertility journey began, I have seen many things, good and bad. I've worn many hats—some have made me grow, and some have made me jaded. It's all been a part of the journey. We didn't come home with the grand biological-baby prize. Instead, we came home with thirty-five thousand dollars in debt—which we've only recently paid off. I'm taking meds to try to reverse the physical damage done to my body, which never fully went back to normal. Mental and emotional damage takes time and patience, and there is no time limit, no matter how much you want to move on. Grief is not linear or predictable.

Sometimes, you need to put boundaries in place for yourself, to protect those still-raw, open wounds. I still can't do baby showers, all these years later. I used to think about it and feel beyond guilty, but now, I just recognize it as my limit. I often send a gift—but that's all I can do. Seeing round bellies and newborn baby things is just too much, and I refuse to let my grief ruin someone else's day or pull me down into the depths again. It is my boundary, and I try very hard not to cross it.

My grief is not linear, and yours isn't, either—no matter what you battle. You don't have to apologize for your grief. You don't have to explain why you can or cannot do things. Guess what I've learned? *No* is a full sentence—and I think we forget that. As women, we are conditioned to say, "No, but . . . ," "No, because . . . ." We must justify our answers, or they are not considered valid. *No* can just be *no*, without having an explanation.

After our infertility journey ended, I thought about all I had endured to make our dream come true. The more I realized what the fertility doctors' "success rate" meant versus reality, I was disgusted. When a fertility clinic shares their "success rate," it is determined by the number of successful positive pregnancy tests they have achieved. However, their true success rate is based on "live births," which is a much lower statistic. With more research, I learned it's known that your first IVF is likely to fail. Some women will do an average of three IVF cycles before pregnancy is achieved. The success rate of IVF goes up with each round, and the odds of success rise the most between six to nine rounds. The

Only the Strong Survive

success rate is still only at 54 percent, which means 46 percent of women are unsuccessful in achieving pregnancy—or their pregnancies end in miscarriage.

I've known other women to go through more than one IVF cycle, and I don't know how they've done it. When you are in it, deep in it, your brain can't break the cycle of *what ifs*. There is always that metaphoric carrot dangling of *maybe this time it will work*, over and over again, until it happens, and you are finally pregnant, you choose to stop, or you break. I broke. Some may say that I knew my limit and I stopped, but I know that, not so deep down, I felt myself shatter.

When you are a patient at a fertility clinic, you are a number that adds to their success rate or not. They want you to succeed for their ratings—not necessarily your benefit. The nurses are amazing and are your support system, but it's the system that is broken when it comes to patient support. Women are pumped full of drugs without second thought. They are put through barbaric procedures with only over-the-counter painkillers in their systems while wide awake. Would they put a man through these things? I'm not sure they would. Most women don't have an outside support system, and they don't feel like they can talk about it openly and honestly with their friends and family, so they suffer alone.

When Ashley agreed to look into adoption, transitioning from the headspace of fertility treatments to adoption wasn't easy. Anyone can walk into a fertility clinic and say, "I want to have a baby." The doctor says, "OK, let's do some tests," and they start the process. Adoption—that's a whole other ballgame. Family and Children Services information nights, PRIDE Training, police checks, home studies, profile books, and waiting for a match. Your whole life is put out there for someone to analyze, and that can really be nerve wracking—especially with everything we had already been through. And when it came to our relationship, we were private people.

Ashley Biddiscombe

We were in for a whole new journey in unknown territory, and it was scary. However, the next steps would change our outlook on life in ways we never imagined.

FOUR:
A New Journey

The adoption information session wasn't long after our last fertility appointment. If we were going to decide if this is what our next step would be, we had might as well know what it was all about sooner than later, and I felt desperate for answers. I just needed something to show me a light at the end of the tunnel.

It was a weeknight. Winter had already overstayed its welcome. You could hear the winter slush under the tires as we pulled into the parking lot of Family and Children Services. We made our way into the newer building. It was empty as we tried to figure out what boardroom we would be in, and I was nervous we had no idea what to expect. We found the large room filled with other couples, and found our chairs. The presenters offered us coffee from the snack table, and I could feel my cheeks warm as I realized how tired I was from the full day of work. I looked around the room and realized we were again the only same-sex couple in the room of about fifteen other couples. We sat down with our coffees and waited.

The next hour was filled with information about various kinds of adoption, information on home studies and children in foster care. We had originally had our sights set on private adoption, but it was becoming clear as the presentation continued that may be a harder road than we thought. With today's advancements in medicine, freedom of choice, and financial aid, not as many women were looking to place infants with prospective birth families. We had thinking to do as we left with a file folder of resources and information to pour over. We chatted lightly on the car ride home. I think we were both afraid of stepping too far in either direction.

A few months later, Ashley looked at me one night as we were sitting in our room.

"I'm OK not having kids. What if it's just the two of us?" I stared at her. Even though I was still fighting through my infertility grief and depression, I was excited at the possibility of adoption and the options it gave us.

"But we've been wanting a family since the beginning. Why would you say that?" I felt a little frantic.

"I don't want kids anymore."

The sentence was short and to the point. There was a hard look behind her eyes—one that I had never seen before.

She had put the brakes on. She didn't want to look into anything, she didn't want kids . . . period. *I had just gone through four years of fertility treatments for her to suddenly not to want kids?* I can't remember exactly what was said after that—all I know is that I was livid—seeing-red kind of livid. There were some nasty words flung around on my end, and crying—I do know that. I slammed our bedroom door and drove to my parents' house for the night. We were at a crossroads. All I wanted was our family—and in that moment, she did not. I cried myself to sleep that night in a bed that wasn't my own. We were both grieving, in different directions. I wasn't going to give up on my dream, and I wasn't giving up on our marriage. So where did that leave us?

We moved around the house in an awkward silence that seemed to linger. When we did talk, we avoided anything that resembled talk about a family, children, or babies. It felt like we were living on two different planets. Nothing felt put together, but like broken little pieces that just weren't fitting the same. We worked, we came home. We smiled and laughed with family and friends, but behind closed doors, the feeling of being a married couple—the "in it together" sense—wasn't there. We just coexisted, for months on end.

One day, we were passing each other in the basement as we did chores and she looked at me out of the blue and said, "Let's try adoption." I stopped dead in my tracks and turned around, staring at her in disbelief.

"Wait, what?!" I didn't think I had heard her right.

"I think we should look into adoption."

"Are you sure? Like really sure?" She nodded. I didn't know why she had changed her mind, but she did. I can tell you that I was on the computer faster than I should have been looking up our next steps.

We had awhile to wait. PRIDE Training dates were booked far in advance, but there was a glimmer of hope back in me that I hadn't felt in a long time. We could take the training through Family and Children Services or privately. We decided to take the training privately. It was more expensive, but there weren't any waitlists, and we could get in sooner. As I looked down the list of trainer's names, my eye looked at one specific name—*Angela*—and my gut said, *fill out the inquiry form*, and I hit send.

We had the summer, fall, and winter to wait, so we put everything in the back of our heads and enjoyed life. We took our niece regularly for sleepovers, and I babysat her most of that summer, doing day trips and enjoying life with a little one in tow. We focused on our families. I focused on my classes at the barn and spoiling my horse. Ashley poured herself into work and growing the business. She had big hopes and dreams, and I wanted to see her to reach them. She had poured so much of herself into our infertility. She could now focus on what she wanted to do without guilt. We went onto live life without the stress of fertility treatments, and we let ourselves try to heal—sometimes, easier said than done.

Finally, April 2015 came along, and it was time for us to start PRIDE Training. "PRIDE" stands for Parent Resources for Information, Development, and Education, which is a twenty-seven-hour educational program to prepare and educate potential foster and adoptive families. Everyone wanting to foster or adopt must complete the program before moving onto the next steps. My first thought was, *Why the heck do we need parental training? How hard can it be?* When you give birth, they hand you the baby and send you home. You don't get training. Man, was I so wrong.

We pulled into the smallest parking lot outside on old downtown building. Us and two other weary couples got out of our cars and headed into the white building. We found ourselves in a small meeting room, greeted by Angela and another trainer. We sat down at the tables formed into a square, where we could see and interact with everyone. I have never been one for big groups, or for raising my hand and participating. Even in school growing up, I was the quiet one, trying not to get called on. This tiny group was my kind of scene—which is funny, because every week, I stood in the arena with six riders and up to eighteen volunteers, and I oversaw them all and never questioned my own abilities. But you're always more comfortable in your home, and the barn was my second home.

We did our introductions, and they handed each of us a three-inch binder filled to the brim with information, and we began. To this day, that binder still sits in the top of our closet, collecting dust, but still tucked away for safe keeping.

The next eight hours flew by. We covered all different aspects of adoption. Sometimes, I can take a while to dive into a new topic—but this had me invested in learning, right from the first hour. We knew we had some heavy topics in the upcoming sessions, but the eye-opening experience was amazing. It felt like a secret world that not many people got to be apart of or fully understood. Ashley and I got home that night and slipped into the hot tub. Though it had been a long day, we couldn't stop talking about what we had just experienced. We were looking forward to going back the next day. For the first time in a long time, I remember feeling excited and genuinely happy again. From cold fertility doctors' offices to this new bright, supportive, information-filled training was a game-changer not only for me, but for us as a couple.

The following weekend was tough-topic time. We covered childhood trauma, drug abuse, sexual abuse, and fetal alcohol syndrome. The other trainer shared her own adoption journey, which was like something you would read in a book—equally heartbreaking and heartwarming. Even though it was a lot to process at times, I felt like I had come home, in a way—and not one ounce of me wanted to back down. I knew in my core I was meant for this path. But what surprised me the most was Ashley, and how she seemed to take it all in stride. For the first time in a long time, I felt the teamwork I didn't know I had been missing. I watched her smile and laugh, and we were talking about the future again, like a dark cloud had been lifted, and we were hand in hand again.

During these training weekend s ,we would have open and honest conversations about what we were willing to take on in a child's profile. Topics such as what age range you would prefer. Would you be willing to take on a child exposed to drugs? Are you open to having an open adoption with birth parents or a birth family? You sit and talk about what you think you can manage in your life as an individual and as a couple. Our list was meek and mild-looking. Some of the tougher topics I still felt like I was too wildly uneducated in to be able to confidently say I could take them on in our home. Even though I had experience with disabilities professionally and personally, Ashley did not, and we had to agree what severity we were willing to take on, if any at all.

The last day ended with real adoptive parents telling us their adoption stories. One woman spoke about going to the ARE and finding her children's profiles there. Angela explained to us during our training earlier that that ARE stood for Adoption Resource Exchange. It is a conference that takes place twice a year, and the Children's Aid Societies (CAS) from all over the province come together for a weekend bringing, all the profiles of their hard-to-place children. Hard-to-adopt profiles tend to be those children who are in their teenage years, sibling groups, and those with disabilities. This allows these profiles to be exposed to any eligible adoptive parent who wants to attend. Normally when adopting through CAS—also known as Family and Children Services—you are restricted to your own region. The ARE gives you the opportunity to look at other regions, outside of your own.

After the adoptive families told their stories, Ashley turned and looked at me, and said point-blank, with conviction, "I want to go to the ARE in November."

I looked at her. "What? Why? None of those cases are what we talked about."

"I know. I want to go, though. I just want to see it." And she was adamant, and I had no idea why.

"OK, we can do that . . . ." I thought it was an impulsive idea, one of those *seemed like a good idea at the time* kind of things, but I would later find out she was serious—dead serious—and according to her, it *had* to be November. Angela looked at us both, laughing to herself, shaking her head.

"You two are totally going to adopt a sibling group." We rolled our eyes at her and laughed her off. Only crazy people adopt more than one child at a time, and a sibling group was not on our list. However, she saw something in us that we didn't see in ourselves—and she knew.

There is something about sharing a new experience with people you've never met before. You walk in guarded and unsure, but leaving, it's almost hard to say goodbye. You have all come together for different reasons, but leave with the same knowledge and experience—like a secret club that no one else can be a part of. I've kept in touch with one of the couples over the years, to see how they made out on their journey. After so much time spent together, you hope that they, too, find what they are looking for, and you cheer them on in whatever they choose, because you are a part of the secret club—and no one else truly knows.

We approached Angela and asked if she would be willing to do our home study for us. A home study is a series of interview sessions lasting one to two hours that does not only screen prospective families, but creates a full profile that is used for adoption matches. Home studies cover family history, medical history, financial history, and your interests. It also includes police checks, CAS checks, a medical report, a house inspection, and references. Your life is basically under a microscope. It's not designed to keep you from making a family, but for making sure they find the right fit for your family. It also keeps children protected—especially those who have already experienced so much in their lives already. Legally, you must have a home study completed before proceeding with fostering or adopting.

Angela was not only a social worker, but she was licensed and specialized in adoptions. Trying to go through Family and Children Services for our home study was going to take longer than we were willing to wait. To us, it was worth the extra money to get it done privately—especially if it was someone we already felt like we had a connection with.

Luckily, Angela agreed. We had to wait a bit to get started, but we were on our way and feeling as confident as we could considering. While we waited, we started collecting paperwork and looking around the house, becoming hyper-aware of every unsafe thing that could potentially kill or maim a child—which is everything, by the way. You've got a stove . . . danger. Stairs . . . danger. Medication you've never thought twice about . . . danger. That alcohol bar you spent years building up for house parties . . . danger. Cleaning supplies . . . danger.

Before the first meeting at our house, I have never in my life panic-cleaned the way I did that week. And I don't mean you clean the morning of your first interview. I mean the kind of manic cleaning when you realize your baseboards haven't been touched since you moved in. I was not going to let anything hinder this assessment. The reference materials said we had to have outlet covers—those little plastic things that keep children from getting electrocuted—and you can guarantee we had those outlet covers, even on the outlets you couldn't see. I wasn't any taking chances. We had to have alcohol in a locked cabinet, fire extinguishers accessible, carbon monoxide detectors, and our water tank a certain temperature. I would've vacuumed the cats if that was a requirement. You go a little crazy all at once. In reality, your first meeting doesn't leave your living room area—or the couch for that matter—but I would be prepared for anything.

However, it isn't anything like what you have in your head, and you are overreacting. Yes, you do have to have all the safety things in place eventually, but the first meetings are for the social worker to get to know you and to make sure you don't have drug needles laying on the floor or your home isn't completely falling apart. She wasn't looking at my freshly scrubbed baseboards. You don't have to have the perfect single detached with large, fenced yard—you just need safe and loving home of any size.

As the next few months passed, we were ticking off all the boxes to get the home study completed. We had interviews together and separately at our home, and at Angela's office. We had our police checks and medicals. We were coming down to the wire before the ARE, but Angela promised we would have it all done. We had to have it to be eligible adoptive parents, and if we found a potential match, but I was still in the mindset that we were just going to see what it was all about.

In November 2015, a week before the ARE, an email package of information arrived that we could scan through before we were to go in person. It contained general adoption information: a list of the children's names, ages, and regions/locations, and information about a log-in we would receive to be able to see the children's profiles and pictures on an online private platform in the upcoming days. I opened the email at home. Ashley opened it at work. We both printed the papers with the children's names and ages. When we compared notes later, we had circled the same children we wanted more information about. We were definitely on the same page.

I was anxious to see the profiles online, but like everything in adoption . . . you wait. Then, finally, the email came, a couple days before we were to leave for Toronto. I sat down at our dining room table, my stomach fluttering slightly. Up until now, everything had been hypothetical and on paper—but there were going to be pictures of actual children living out there in the world, in foster homes, waiting for their forever families. I took a deep breath and opened the log-in. Little faces were staring back at me in profile pictures. So many tiny humans, of all ages and races, needing a family to call their own, at no fault of their own. When excitement takes over, but then hit with the heaviness that is reality of why these children are in foster care, it can be extremely overwhelming. You feel like if you choose to look at one profile over another one, you're doing disservice to the ones you aren't looking at. You battle with the idea of *why isn't that child worthy of me looking at their information?*

I was scrolling away when I stopped, I clicked, and I saw them. Two blonde-haired, blue-eyed toddlers. In that moment, I instantly thought, *Those are my kids.* I don't know what it was, but it almost took my breath away. I quickly shoved those thoughts down as deep as I could, but they kept bubbling up, like boiling water. Their profile was heavy, but still erred on the side of caution with the information given. There was video attached, and I watched them come to life on the screen. The boy looked under a year old. His hair was longer and curled around his neck, and he wore a little blue plaid shirt. The little girl was playing blocks, trying to stack them. She had a sass to her, and I'm pretty sure the video cut out right before she let out a scream. I sat, a little stunned at myself, as I stared at them. *You can't know right away, right? That seems silly, and there is no way I am getting my hopes up about this. I can't crash and fall again. My psyche can't take it.* I closed my computer and tried to move on with my day. But I would log in again . . . more times than I want to admit.

Ashley came home that night from work and asked, "Did you look at the profiles online?" I told her I had. Neither of us were quite ready to say how we were really feeling.

"There's definitely some I'd like to know more about," she said loosely, and I nodded in agreement, trying to be casual about it—but I was anxious.

Only days later, we were in the Jeep, heading toward Toronto to a hotel and conference centre. We parked the car and headed in to find the table to register. The conference was being held in a huge ballroom on the second level. We gave our names and information and were handed a package before we headed upstairs. I think I held my breath all the way up the escalator. We took an extra moment to take our coats off and get organized before heading through one of the many doors leading in.

The room was filled with long tables and display boards. Aisles separated the regions. It was similar-looking to a job or volunteer fair. Each region had their own area with display boards. All the pictures we had seen online covered the display boards. Underneath each picture were names and ages. On the tables, there was information from that CAS, and different medical conditions you may not be familiar with that were associated with their children. Volunteers stood and sat by the tables, waiting to be asked any questions regarding a specific profile.

In the far-back hallway, there was a room where you could sit and watch videos of each child that was being profiled. Another room was a dedicated break room, if you just needed to sit to breathe or talk privately. It was a very overwhelming place to walk into for the first time. But we were here to learn and ask questions, so we started to move around the room.

I did my best to keep my head focused, but all I could think about was finding those two little faces. We took our time and went region to region, looking at the display boards. Then we came down one of the middle aisles, and there they were. The table was surrounded by couples, and my heart sank a little. But when you have a sibling group of younger children who were stinking adorable, how could you not expect it to be busy? We really wanted to talk to the social worker. *Patience*, I told myself. *It's not like someone is going to scoop them up and take them home. They aren't here.* We walked around to look at the other profiles, and would head back when it was not as busy.

We stopped a booth that was for a region just outside of our own. A little boy, about six years old, had caught our eye while we had been looking at the online profiles. We talked to the social worker briefly, filled out the application, and handed it into the worker. We had put our names forward for the first time for an actual child. I should have felt more overwhelmed by the act of filling out that form, but my brain was elsewhere.

Down another aisle, there was a toddler, just over a year old. She was beautiful, with little strawberry-blonde curls. The worker told us that she had a genetic disorder, and that her life expectancy was only a few short years, and that they were looking for a home that could love her in her remaining time. After all that we had been through already, could we bring a child into our home knowing we only had limited time with her, and then watch her die? My heart ached at the idea, and ached more for the fact I didn't think I could handle it.

In another region, there was a little girl who had long, brown hair with bangs and blue eyes. She was deaf and had autism. I was very drawn to her profile, but Ashley said that would be too much to take on for her, and I had I knew I had to respect that. I've thought about that little girl now and then over the years. Her picture has taken up residence in my brain. I don't know why she sits with me more than any other profile we passed up. Part of me still wishes we would've put our names forward. I hope they all found families that weekend.

Most of the crowd had dispersed around the other table, and we headed back over. There were still about five couples all wanting information ,and the social worker gave us all the overview at the same time. The case was just as heavy in person as it had been online—a sibling group, both with disabilities. The diagnosis was unknown at the time, but there was suspected global developmental delay in the little girl, but little blonde-haired boy with curls future was still unknown. As the worker spoke, we watched the couples walk away, until we were the only ones left. I stepped forward and asked the disability-specific questions I wanted to ask, and she answered what she could.

We stepped aside and chatted. "I want to put an application in," I said. And to my surprise Ashley turned to me and said, "So do I". These two little humans were the complete opposite of what we had written down on our list during our PRIDE training, but the driving force we both had towards this profile was something we couldn't explain. What I had felt when I first saw their profiles, Ashley had, too. We handed over our application, and the worker said they would be looking at everything within two weeks.

We had both done what we had set out to do, and walked out of the conference room and back to the Jeep. All we could do then was wait. And Ashley will tell you I am not the kind of person who waits patiently.

FIVE:
On the Other Side of the Door

When we had started the adoption process, we were prepared for it to take a while. We had settled into the idea it could take a couple of years after our home study was completed—but there we were, invested in two little humans that we did not even know, less than three months later.

Two weeks came and went, then I received a call from Angela.

"The agency called. They think they may have a potential match in their own region. They are going to look at that lead first. They had thirty-one applications—there was a lot of interest." My heart sank. "I'll call you if anything changes."

I hung up and called Ashley. I knew I shouldn't have gotten my hopes up—my gut had been wrong. I retold her what Angela had said, and without missing a beat, she said, "It's all going to work out. I'm not worried. Those are our kids."

At first, I thought she was just trying to keep my hopes up. But she was serious, and was not worried at all. I shook my head and hung up the phone, and had a little cry. I shouldn't have gotten my hopes up. I should've known better after all these years. Nothing came easy for us.

Ashley Biddiscombe

I always seemed to be in the car when Angela called, and two weeks later was no different. I saw her number pop up. I put her on speakerphone as I was driving to work.

"The match backed out. They are opening it back up to ARE applications. It's between you and another couple." I don't even know if I had a chance to say, *Hi, how are you?*

"Are you serious?" I pulled over into a parking lot.

I could hear her excitement in her voice. "Yeah—and I think you have a good chance—but I need to ask again: are you sure this is what you want? This is nothing like we talked about at all. This is a complicated profile."

"We are completely sure."

"OK. I will let them know, they want to make sure they have the best match. I will keep you posted."

I hung up that phone and called Ashley, trying to keep my shit together.

"We are back in! It didn't work out. They are looking at us and another couple, Angela said . . . "

In almost a creepy, but calm tone, Ashley said, "Those are our kids. It's all going to work out."

Has something possessed you? How are you so calm about all of this? Like seriously. I had the jitters for days.

It was a sunny December day, blue skies—and the first snowfall had yet to cover the grass, which still made it feel like fall. I was driving to the barn to see my horse when the phone rang. I looked down saw Angela's phone number, and right then, knew . . . .

"They are yours . . . . The other couple backed out, and CAS thinks you are a good fit. I don't know all the details yet . . . ."

I think I blocked out the conversation after *they are yours..* I called Ashley, and she answered, laughing.

"I told you. It's about time. So, now what happens?" *It's about time . . . pssh.* I shook my head. She had been so legitimately convinced this was happening the whole time that this wasn't even surprising news to her.

We would have to wait until the new year to get any more information. We would spend Christmas with our families, and update them on all that had happened. And as I sat beside the Christmas tree on Christmas Eve, that warm, twinkle-light glow filling the living room, I sipped mulled wine, and I couldn't help but to think, *This is our last Christmas without children . . . . Next year, we will have kids to celebrate with. I wonder what that will look like?* I looked around at our family, and at Ashley, and smiled, soaking everything in.

We had a scheduled call with the kid's social worker, case worker, and foster mom, as well as Angela, in February 2016. Ash and I sat on our couch with our pens and paper ready. All the questions we had were about to have answers. Ashley, being clever, also used her phone to record the call, so we could relisten to it if we needed to.

This was a no-fluff kind of call. We were going to hear all the details about the kids. The good and bad—about their disabilities, behaviours, some of their history—basically, a make-it-or-break-it call, all out on the table. We heard about an already-failed adoption, and them wanting to be sure this time. They had many services and specialists in place already that could be transferred to our region. My choppy notes read . . .

Felicia, three years old, was just starting some self-care, like dressing herself, though she was still in a crib for her own safety and for Chase's—she liked to pull his arms through the bars. Not out of diapers yet . . .

- *Has to duct-tape her diaper on, put a bathing suit on, a onesie and a sleep sack to keep her from smearing feces all over the room.*
- *She self-harmed by scratching, biting, or banging her head.*

Ashley Biddiscombe

- *She is a climber, so furniture in her room must be limited.*
- *Does not transition well and tests all boundaries.*
- *Tore through three crib mattresses with her bare hands... is this kid the Hulk?*

Looking back on our notes as I write, this one line made me laugh: *Communicates through high-pitched scream while outside of the home. It isn't always when she is frustrated—now, when she screams there seems to be more of a purpose to it.* We will talk more about this later.

I remember looking at Ashley. "She has autism. Do they not know she has autism?" This little girl needed all the help she could get.

Chase, eighteen months old...
- *Preemie born at twenty-eight weeks, blind until he was eight months old, still being monitored.*
- *Low muscle tone, and just starting to sit on his own in the last few months, but has also started crawling.*
- *Does not cope well in new environments. It's very overwhelming.*
- *Slept almost twenty hours a day until he was five months old*
- *Just started eating solid foods, but still on formula.*
- *Needs more medical intervention to determine his function and future.*

Now, if you've made it this far into the list, I am sure you are thinking, *Oh my God, this is a lot.* Our notes from this call are three pages long—and it was a lot. Angela was questioning our decision when we said goodbye to the others on the call. Ashley and I looked at each other and said, "We can do this." We were determined to bring our children home. We would be waiting for more information on next steps in the months to come.

Only the Strong Survive

Our first trip was in April 2016. We drove six hours up to meet our children for the first time. Even though I have family in that area, we stayed in a hotel. We needed somewhere to breathe; this was about to be a lot. We were both anxious in our own ways. Media likes to give you a visual expectation about foster care and adoption. It's really hard to imagine what you will be stepping into for your first time.

We were going to meet with the social worker and case worker the next morning for breakfast, before heading to the foster home. We arrived in the city that evening, checked into our hotel, had some food, crawled into the bed, and didn't sleep. A) obviously we were nervous; b) I'm pretty sure the people in the room next to us were having a hotel party, which kept us up most of the night, despite our calls to the front desk.... Not the way we planned on spending the night.

We got up the next morning with bags under our eyes. The sun was shining, and it was clear-blue skies—the perfect spring day—as we headed to the restaurant. When I get nervous, I get lightheaded and jittery. Lack of sleep didn't help. I had to put my logical brain on and try to act normal—whatever *normal* was before you met your children for the first time. A lot easier said than done. We pulled up in the parking lot, took one last, deep breath, and headed inside.

The restaurant was busy, and two lovely blonde ladies and an older lady who I didn't recognize from all our other interactions greeted us, and we sat down. I later found out the extra body was the head of the adoption section at CAS. I think she wanted to meet the two crazy people willing to look at this case. Felicia and Chase were one of the hardest placements they had, and everyone wanted to make sure this was it. I almost felt like child playing the part as an adult as I sat down. I needed coffee and food. We didn't know what the day was going to look like, and as nervous as I was, I couldn't let my hypoglycemia make an entrance, too. Nothing

47

says "we are capable, give your children to us" better than passing out from not taking care of yourself in front of CAS workers.

We ordered our food and got down to business as they filled us in more about the process and what the day was all about. I think I comprehended most of it, but at times, I felt like I was living someone else's life. Halfway through our meal, Ashley got up and left the table. I found out later, when we were alone, that she had puked her guts out in the bathroom. Anxiety was high. We finished at the restaurant, and we were all loading into cars to meet at the foster home to finally meet our children.

We pulled up in front of a simple townhouse. Kids' toys were on the front porch. Nothing special or scary about this place. No one was singing "It's a Hard Knock Life." We got out of the car and started to walk up the driveway. The social worker knocked on the front door, and just like that, time stood still for a moment.

Six years ago, almost to the day, we had sat in the fertility clinic for the first time. There was one last door to go through, and what we had been waiting for was waiting for us on the other side. This was it, and suddenly, my jitters were completely gone. I forced the tears welling up in my eyes back down as the door opened.

Melissa, the kids' foster mom, opened the door with a cheery "hello," her curly hair bouncing as she moved, and we walked in. Within three seconds, a little tiny body hopped off the couch, ran over to Ashley, and asked to be picked up. Ashley was holding our daughter. She was in a pink, plaid shirt, and her little scrawny legs were in leggings. She was fearless, and I think in that moment, Felicia stole a tiny piece of Ash's heart. Ashley carried her into the living room, and the little, blonde-haired boy who no longer had his long curls was on his tummy on the floor, playing with a firetruck, wearing a baby blue polo shirt and navy blue pants. He was much smaller than I imagined—only around size of a nine-month-old. His little, tiny feet were in baby socks, and he was scooting his body across the floor so he could hit the fire truck

Only the Strong Survive

and watch it roll away. It was hard to believe that they were three and nineteen months old—they were so tiny. All our waiting was finally done, and here they were. That big, scary list from the call months earlier looked extremely different in person.

We spent the day interacting with the kids and talking with Melissa and the social workers, getting a feel for daily life. It's really weird interacting with your children, who you know nothing about, in front of the people who have been protecting them since birth. The social workers said goodbye and left us in Melissa's care for the rest of the afternoon. Before we left for dinner and the night, Melissa said, "OK, let's get a picture!" and before I could comprehend what was going on, we had two kids in our arms, and we had our first family picture taken. We headed back to the hotel exhausted, but couldn't stop talking about all that had happened.

The next day, we met Melissa and the kids at a petting farm before we were going to start our journey home. We were basically going to see the kids in the wild, and interact with them how we would naturally. Melissa had brought along two of her own children as well—a little boy that was the same age as Felicia and an older daughter. We walked around the farm and played on the playground. Felicia wanted to do what she wanted to do, and "no" was merely a suggestion in her world. She was active but happy. Chase was in the stroller, happy to be along for the ride, but you could not stop moving, or he would cry. We took turns with the kids, trying to get in equal time and bond.

As I was walking with Felicia—wait, let's be honest, we were running, Felicia, as quick as a kid can be, grabbed a water bottle out of a stranger's stroller and promptly put it in her mouth. I went to tell her, "No, that's not ours" and take it back from her, but before I could blink, her teeth were clamped around my finger—that little bugger bit me as hard as she could, and refused to let go. The only thing I could think to do was blow air directly in her face, in hopes she would let go, and pray she didn't pull back.

Ashley Biddiscombe

Thankfully, she did let go—and then off she ran, tossing the water bottle to the ground. All I could think was, *You little shit*. Ah—kind thoughts of a new mother. I needed a moment to regroup. We traded kids, and I took the stroller for a walk. I stopped for a moment and took Chase out, since he wouldn't stop crying. I stood in the shade and rocked him back and forth, bouncing, and with that, he instantly fell asleep—and stayed asleep if I was moving. I watched Ashley pushing Felicia and her foster brother on a big tire swing in the distance, as happy as can be.

We said our goodbyes in the parking lot and headed back to the highway toward home. I turned to Ashley as we drove.

"She bit me." I held up my purple, still-dented finger.

Ashley started to laugh. "What? When?"

"Before you took them to the tire swing. I tried to take a bottle away, and she bit me."

By this point, Ashley was dying of laughter. "I guess we better watch for that, eh? She's like a tiny piranha."

I couldn't help but laugh, too. Not quite the sweet first moments you expect to have with your daughter.

We would be making this twelve-hour round trip almost every weekend. We would work Monday to Friday, leave Friday night, and get home late before starting work on Monday. We would spend Saturday and Sunday, breakfast until bedtime with the kids, going on outings, doing day to day routines, feeding, changing, baths, and putting them to bed before driving home the six hours on Sunday night. We would do this for almost three months.

When we were home, we were preparing. Bedrooms needed to be painted, and finishing touches to be completed. I went shopping for cribs and dressers with my mom, and when they arrived, my parents came over to help. It's hard enough putting one crib together, and we had two. Baby gates had to be installed, and we had to rearrange the living rooms for all the new toys we had acquired. Cabinets were rearranged to fit bottles and plastic toddler dishes, and two highchairs were sat in the dining room. When you go from two adults to two parents and two toddlers, the house fills very quickly—especially when you need two of everything.

SIX:
Coming Home

As we approached June, as a collective, we decided to transition the kids home, one at a time. We would start with Chase, believing it would be an easier transition on him than Felicia. The thought of this being the second-last twelve-hour round trip was starting to sound rather good around this time. Ashley was going to take a parental leave with me until the kids were settled. The house was ready, and so were we. Just as we had done on every other trip, we loaded up and hit the road. We didn't pack a bag this time. It was a round trip. We had been on the road for a few hours when a call came in.

"It's Melissa. Chase is sick. I thought it was just a basic cold, but it's getting bad. I'm worried. We are heading to the Children's Hospital. I don't know if he will be able to go home this weekend. It's up to you if you decide to still come." I looked at Ash and she nodded.

"No, we are coming. We will be there in a few hours."

"OK. When you get into town, meet us at the hospital. I will let them know you are coming."

And we hung up. We drove as fast as legally and not-so-legally as we could the next three hours, without stopping. Melissa sent us pictures of our little man in his carrier, oxygen mask on, his little chubby arm attached to a board, all taped up, with his IV in. She texted me a small update and told us where to go once we arrived.

Once we arrived, we navigated our way through the emergency room and found them in a decent-sized room with a glass door.
"They think it's RSV. They have been giving him breathing treatments, but his fever isn't breaking. He's one sick little dude." Melissa looked down at him in his car seat carrier.
Nurses bustled about, checking him regularly. We watched the time pass, and he wasn't getting any better. The doctor came back in.
"We must admit him until this fever breaks and his breathing improves. The meds don't seem to be working yet. It'll be a bit, but we will be moving him upstairs in a little while." We nodded. I felt like a fish out of water suddenly. What did all this mean?
Melissa turned to us, shaking her curl-filled hair. "I can't stay. I have to get back to the kids at home, I've called CAS and I've talked to the hospital. You guys are so close to signing these papers that they've agreed that you can stay with him as his parents. Are you ok with that?"
"Yes of course we will stay." I look up at her. What was I going to say? No, we would just abandon him here with a volunteer caregiver?
"OK, I am going to run home and grab containers of formula and his things. You will have enough for tonight, and I will be back in the morning. Keep me posted if anything changes." I nodded slowly, looking at Ashley, who was standing, rocking him. He looked so small and so sick. And just like that Melissa left, we were alone with an extremely sick boy.

If you've ever had a child in an emergency room, time feels like it moves at a snail pace. We sat, rocked, and paced, as nurses came in to check on him. The doctor came in and let us know it would still be a bit before he would be moved, and only one parent could go upstairs with him. We agreed I would. Ashley would call Angela to tell her what was going on. And she was determined to turn around and drive home to pack bags and come back.

"You're going to drive all the way home *tonight*?" I looked at her as she stood holding Chase, the IV pole close by, his bare little chest against hers.

"We don't have anything with us. We need clothes. I need to organize the animals and work at home. We don't know what will happen—and let's just be prepared. I will leave tonight and drive back up first thing in the morning. I'll be fine. I'm not tired. I'll sleep when I get home. Traffic will be nothing at this time at night."

We were running on pure adrenaline as we said goodbye, and Ashley was back on the road. Then, just like that, it was just me and my little boy.

We turned the lights off and I sat down in the chair. His hot little body was asleep on my chest as I breathed him in and stroked his hair, he still smelled like baby. This was not how I was expecting our first parenting experience to go, that's for sure. Both feet into the deep end. There was no way I was moving. This little man needed sleep, and for the first time ever, I was completely alone with him. I was happy to soak that in. It was about 10 p.m., when I heard a familiar voice come down the hallway. I looked up and my uncle was standing in the doorway in his police uniform. My mom had called him.

He smiled. "The uniform gets you into places. The nurses let me back." I was floored, and beyond thankful to see a familiar face.

"Meet Chase," I glanced down at his pale, sleeping face. He was in only his diaper, to try to get his fever down—oxygen in his nose and IV in his arm. "We thought we would make things interesting." I smiled, shrugging. He stayed with me for an hour or so before I gave him one last, big hug, and we were alone again, with only the sounds and glow of the nurse's station outside the glass door.

The nurse came in a little while later to tell us we were finally moving upstairs. I put Chase into the stroller Melissa had left. I pushed while the nurse followed behind with his IV pole. We weaved through the hospital until we found the elevator, and up we went.

"The rooms in isolation are pretty big. You'll have your own bathroom," the nurse said quietly as we moved through the dimly lit hallways. I don't think I fully comprehended what "you're being admitted" meant when the doctor had said it originally—and then it hit me as we got off on the "isolation floor." We were in our own room. The first door went into a wash area, the second into the actual room. His big, metal hospital crib was in one space close to the door. There was a chair that folded down into a bed tucked under the far window, and an extra rocking chair, and a full bathroom. The room was huge—but this was a lot worse than I thought. When they had said he was sick, they hadn't been lying.

The nurse hooked him up to heart monitors. His oxygen was taped to his face as he kept grabbing at it, and they had to redo his IV for a second time because he ripped it out. He was scared, and I was scared, then, as they added more tubes and monitors, which were on either side of the bed, and I could no longer pick him up. I stood over him and ran my fingers along his cheeks until he fell asleep. The nurses came in every half hour to check on him. He was now coughing until he could not breathe, and his fever refused to break. It was one in the morning by the time I was able to pick up my phone and text everyone with updates. I laid my head back in the rocking chair and listened to his raspy breathing and the monitors going on and off. I wasn't going to sleep, and I needed to make sure my wife made it home safely. She pulled in our driveway six hours away at around four o'clock in the morning.

Ashley Biddiscombe

Ashley came into the hospital the next morning. She literally slept for a couple of hours and drove back. I shook my head at her, but she felt like she was doing something to help, and I was so thankful for clean clothes. We had called my aunt, who wasn't too far away. She was going to let us use her house as our crash spot, so we could rotate shifts and get sleep. Our room had a few special privileges. When you are in isolation, it's normally a parent-only zone. But because of our unique situation—we were a couple signatures away from being the parents. Melissa was still foster mom and CAS was still the children's guardian, so they were all allowed in to check on us. I can imagine what I looked like when they walked into the room.

There were no major changes to his condition. We weren't going anywhere anytime soon. He seemed brighter, and drank half a bottle. I was getting rather good at warming the formula in the bathroom sink, and we had a system for weighing his diapers, so the nurses could monitor his in- and output. His case worker insisted she would stay with him so we could get settled at my aunts. Ashley needed sleep after her drive, and I would shower and come back. The look the case worker had in her eyes said she needed the time to sit with him and say goodbye. This would be the last time she would see him before he went home. I smiled and nodded as I closed the door quietly, and I watched a tear run down her cheek as she held him.

The next night wasn't much better. He was on a fair amount of medication, which helped keep the cough from rattling his tiny chest—which also helped him sleep more soundly—but the fever was spiking again. He wasn't happy about the IV, and pulled it again—and he was sick of being poked and prodded. He cried, and at points, he screamed. My heart ached for him. I couldn't move him out of his crib, so I put the sides down and climbed up onto the bed with him, and rocked and whispered to him. Every baby wants their mom when they are sick and fussy, and to him,

I was not it—he wanted Melissa. She was the only mother he knew, and I wasn't cutting it this night. I desperately wanted to be enough for him. In the wee hours of the morning, he finally fell asleep, and I crawled onto the hard bed chair and fell asleep for a couple of hours. I must have slept deeply; I didn't hear the nurses come in for their usual half-hour rounds.

We traded off the next day, and Ashley came to sit with him while I went to my aunts to sleep. I was desperate for a good few hours of sleep on a bed that didn't feel like concrete, and I could roll over and fall off of. I woke up feeling better—not great, but better. I ate food that wasn't food from the hospital cafeteria and headed back to the hospital. I walked into Ashley rocking him quietly in the rocking chair. There were fewer machines attached to him, which was a good sign. The following night was better. He wasn't gasping for air, and his cough was still phlegmy. We had moved onto basic puffers, which I had to give him every few hours. Things were looking a little more normal, and his fever was coming down. I woke up in my bed chair the next morning, and he was standing in this crib, looking around and hungry. I took a picture of him standing in that crib, smiling at me, and I sent it to everyone. We were finally out of the woods.

We were discharged later that day with a bag full of medication. He was going was going back to Melissa's house to be with his foster family for the last night before we would pick him up to head home the following day. I was shocked they were going to let him travel so soon after being discharged, but they insisted he was just fine and could make the trip. After all we had been through those last few days, watching Melissa load him into her van was a lot harder than I had expected. I knew we'd have him the following morning, but I wouldn't have my baby boy that night, and it suddenly felt like part of me was missing.

After a well-deserved full night's sleep, we headed over to Melissa's to meet with the case worker to sign our papers, which would give us guardianship while on adoption probation. Adoption probation lasts a year before you can file your official adoption finalization papers with the court. Melissa took a picture of us while we signed our adoption papers at her dining room table. On a day that should have been filled with excitement and happiness, we look like we had been through an apocalypse. The drained look on my face, and the black circles under my eyes. Ashley looked like she was getting bad news. I chuckle at that picture every time I see it.

Melissa wanted the goodbyes to be quick and short. Chase was her baby, and this was hard on her. I can't even imagine the grief she went through during all of this. To raise a baby from seven weeks old fresh out of the NICU to nineteen months, thinking they may never find their family, and then to watch him drive away. My heart hurts thinking about it. To this day, I consider Melissa one of the most amazing humans I have had the pleasure of knowing. She's a mom and an advocate. She works tirelessly to bring education and support to other parents. If you look up superhuman in the dictionary, I am sure it's her face smiling back.

Ashley loaded the car with Chase's things. Boxes of toys, clothes—his favourite things were coming home with him. Then, just like that, he was in his car seat, and we waved goodbye. We were finally going home.

We were making great time until we were about three hours into the trip. Chase promptly puked all over himself and the Jeep. The multiple days on steroids weren't agreeing with him at all, and in all good-parent fashion, we had to pull over into a parking lot and strip him down. In that moment, I realized the importance of having extra of everything in the car, and that wet wipes were God's gift to parents.

When we finally pulled into the driveway, I had never been so happy to be home—not to mention, in my own bed. We had part of our family home and it was finally time we could do things in our own house, and in our own time. We wouldn't be letting anyone in to meet Chase. He was still sick, and we needed time to ourselves to bond and for him to settle. Felicia was scheduled to come home two weeks later. We wanted a solid base before we added another little body into the mix. However, the next two weeks didn't go smoothly. Having a little boy detoxing off meds and steroids was horrible. He felt so crummy as he screamed and cried, more than should be humanly possible. He puked up every bottle, and he was looking for Melissa to comfort him, and she wasn't there. He was stuck with these two newbies, who clearly weren't doing anything right, in a home that he didn't know.

We decided that we needed more time before bringing Felicia home. It wouldn't be fair to her to come home to this, and we were struggling. By week three, things had calmed down—but loading Chase into the car for a six-hour drive wasn't ideal, since he was just getting settled. CAS allowed us to sign our paperwork remotely, and Ashley called her brother to make the drive with her to pick up Felicia. Felicia wasn't great in the car at all for us. She tended to scream and fuss while you were driving, and I don't mean a scream now and then—I'm talking full-out, top-of-your-lungs screaming, nonstop. For a six-hour drive, she was going to need backup. They did a round trip in a day, and Felicia screamed all the way home, like we had predicted. When they rolled back into the driveway, the Jeep was filled to the brim with the kids' things, including a trampoline—and to this day, I don't know how Ash got it all in.

That night, we laid in our bed. Both children were asleep in their new rooms, and we looked at each other, exhausted. But we had done it. Our family, which we had spent almost six years trying to create, was finally together.

SEVEN:
Not for the Faint of Heart

The first year was the hardest year of my life.

Seems like a bold statement considering everything we had been through up until then. This was a different kind of hard—the emotional, mental, and physical strain was unlike I had ever experienced in my life. I honestly don't know how I didn't drop from stress and exhaustion. When you think about how adoption is portrayed in movies, it looks magical and full of happiness, with smiling kids and smiling parents. The movie *Instant Family* came out in 2018, with Mark Wahlberg and Rose Byrne. I thought this was made by someone who *got it*. It still had its comedy twist, but the bones of the movie were the adoption experience—except in Canada, we don't do the big picnic with children running around, we do the ARE. The struggles, the "what did we do?" conversations in bed, the hairbrush in the toilet—except for us, it was a toothbrush down the sink, the foster and adoptive parent support groups . . . it's all there. I look back at home videos of us and just see shells of two parents trying to make it through. It's like watching a movie of someone else's life.

When Felicia came home, Ashley didn't have a choice but to go back to work. She was supposed to be off on parental leave for longer, but when you own a business, sometimes it's tough to juggle it all. So, it was two toddlers and me during the day . . . all day . . . alone. Felicia, who I often refer to as "The Volcano," had eruptions all day long, and that screaming that they referred to in the original adoption call had made its full appearance every time she didn't get her way—and her way was *never* my way. She would throw her toys, her food. She never walked, she ran. She would dump toys and keep going. She pushed all the boundaries, and she was aggressive—we will talk about that more later. Other times, we would go into her room, and she would be laying down, staring through the bars of her crib, silent tears streaming down her cheeks. She wouldn't look at us or acknowledge our presence. She was depressed, grieving her family. And everything was overwhelming—her entire world had been turned upside down.

Chase was still coming down off his medications. He screamed and cried most of the time, and was never content. His separation anxiety was extreme. He had to be touching me or have the ability to touch me at all times. If I went through our French doors in our hallway to put a laundry basket away, he would sit on the other side with his face pressed up against the glass, scream-crying until he was almost gasping or puking. It was always two seconds too long. His acid reflux was on high tilt. Every bottle that went in came right back up all over him, the floor, or anything in his vicinity. And then there was the sound he made. I can't even fully describe it or mimic it. It was a prominent high-pitched, raspy grunt, and he made it all day long. It was his only way of communicating his frustrations—and *everything* made him frustrated. Anyone who heard it, still refers to it: "Remember that sound Chase used to make?" It clearly made an impression.

Angela says it was one of the worst home transitions she had ever seen—and she had helped many people adopt before us. For the first few months, she was seeing us once a week, just to check in. I am sure she was as worried as we were exhausted. We sat in an adoption support group, and everyone was talking about what they were going through—the ups and downs, successes and failures. Couples talked about the "honeymoon phase" from when their children first came home—and how now it was over, and they had new challenges that they were facing. We never got the "honeymoon phase"—it was hard right from the start.

There weren't any safe daytime activities that I could do alone with the children outside of our home. Even in our home, we were contained to the upper level. It wasn't safe for them to have access to the whole house. Felicia was a runner and climber, and had zero safety skills or awareness. She always needed your full attention, and she didn't transition well—especially in public. Chase wasn't mobile. He had to be carried everywhere, as babies do, which was hard when you needed two hands for both children. I would take the kids in the backyard. Chase hated the feeling of grass touching him, so he would sit on the blanket, throwing toys, and Felicia would look like she was drowning in the kiddie pool as she rolled around in the freezing cold hose water. But they were contained, and happyish. If we weren't in the backyard, we were walking . . . . We did so much walking. We had a double stroller that fit both kids and was my saviour. There were days I just needed out of the house and to look at something different than our four walls. When we were walking, they weren't screaming—and I just needed the screaming to stop. Except the time the stroller wheel slipped on a muddy patch down by the creek in the forest close to our house. I ended up standing knee-deep in the creek, holding up the double stroller with both kids in it . . . that day, I think we were all screaming.

One day, I got brave and stopped at our neighbourhood park. We had been to the park many times when we were doing our trips to Melissa's, but Ashley was always with me to tag team the kids. It was quiet, with only one other family there playing. I thought if I could let Felicia run and keep Chase in the stroller, then it would be manageable. All was going somewhat well, until it was time to go home. I gave her the two-minute warning, and she started instantly screaming. I tried to redirect with the promise of snacks, but she wasn't having it.

"Nooooooo, goooooo!!!!" she screamed, and her body wriggled out of my hands, and she started to run back to the slides. Chase instantly started crying in the stroller. I was too far from him again. I caught my daughter mid-flight as she flailed and swung at me. There was a way you had to hold onto Felicia while she melted down. The goal was to protect her from herself and protect yourself from the scratching, biting, and head-banging. Most of the time, she got me, one way or another. I put her into "the hold," and the flailing turned into kicking, and louder, longer screaming, as I stumbled across the field back to the stroller. I had one chance to get her in and buckled up. It had to be smooth and fast, as I protected my face from her tiny, angry hands. I somehow got her in, and the belt clipped together. She continued to scream like someone was murdering her for the full fifteen-minute walk home. I was exhausted, sweaty, and close to tears. We couldn't even go to the park and be happy. Those moments make you never want to leave the safety of the house again.

In the early days, I was horrified when we made scene. It was loud, aggressive, we stuck out like a sore thumb, and everybody stared. My daughter had no coping skills at all, and she was overstimulated very easily. Unless I had help, I was hesitant to try new things. New environments felt too unknown, too overstimulating, and too hard to do on my own. We were so isolated in our own little chaotic world. I had hopes and dreams of mommy-and-me groups, swimming, and library days. Now, all those places felt impossible.

Ashley would get home from work to find me at my wits' end. We would make dinner, and the kids would eat their portion and ask for more before we could even sit down at the table. For children who were so tiny, they ate adult-sized portions and *more*. As we would get their second helping and then reach for our own, we would realize we didn't make enough for all of us, yet again. Too tired to make more, we would sit down and have the scraps, or not eat at all. Between chasing, meltdowns, walking, and not eating enough, we were exhausted, and at our lowest weights we had been in years. We would collapse into bed at night, and when I would wake up in the morning, Ashley would go to work, and I would lay there, trying to convince myself that I had to get up. I was the only one there to take care of them during the day. I dreaded opening my eyes before forcing myself out of bed. My body felt like a two-tonne weight. I would crawl into the bathroom and look at my black, strained eyes in the mirror before standing in the shower, trying to prepare for another fun day of parental battle. This was not the fairy tale I had imagined. This was beyond hard, and there were days I didn't like the children who I had fought so hard for—but I couldn't admit that to anyone, because this is what we had wanted.

I found Ashley spending more time at work. The days were longer, and she would often not come home until after the children went to bed. She was struggling in a different way than I was, but we didn't really acknowledge it. We were both just trying to get through.

Angela's visits were still at our house, once a month, to do her check-in. I'm sure when she looked at us, she saw the shadows of the people we had been just a few months before. We would talk honestly about our struggles, and she was one of the few we could be honest with about how bad it was. She would remind us we were doing the best we could, and tell us the changes she would see in the kids—even the smallest good changes meant something. To have that outsider looking in was our saving grace. It gave us a reset like nothing else could.

A month after we brought both children home, we had a beach vacation planned. It had been booked well before we even started our trips to visit the kids, and we weren't backing out. Ashley and I were desperate to spend time with our friends. We needed something that felt "normal." We had always brought our niece—who was five at the time—and we did not want her to miss out on the trip. She was adjusting to not having us around as much. We had gone from the fun aunts to Felicia and Chase's moms. Like two crazy people, we loaded up all three children into the truck—two car seats and a booster seat, all lined up. I'm pretty sure the entire house was packed in the bed of the truck. We headed to the cottage to meet our friends.

Chase and Felicia were still in cribs at home. We had gotten playpens for the trip. They *had* to be contained at night, for their safety and our sanity—especially in a new place. We had the camera monitors, and had brought safety locks for the doors, just in case Felicia climbed out and got loose. We knew the cottage from previous trips, and knew that our niece could fit on a cot at the end of our bed for the week—and she was excited to have us to herself at night. Our friend Jill's two children were about the same age as ours, and it was toy central—you name the children's item, we had it. We could do this . . . we could do anything. I think we had to prove that we could still make this trip work to ourselves. It was the one thing we looked forward to every year. We felt like we had lost all sense of normal already, and we couldn't lose this, too.

When you birth children, you know that all their experiences are determined by what you do as a family. When you adopt children, what is "normal" in your life is not in theirs—everything is new. And the beach was one of those experiences. Felicia had experienced a small beach with her foster family, but it was on a tiny lake in a conservation area—not like the large Great Lake we were about to see.

We decided to take all the children on a walk to check out the beach. I had invested in a baby carrier for my back. If Chase was attached to me, he was happy, and wasn't crying, and it left my hands free to catch the wild child. It was perfect. I loaded him up onto my back. My niece and one of Jill's girls held hands as they chatted away, like little girls do, and Ashley had Felicia. We walked down the set of stairs to the sand, and I turned around just in time to see Felicia's face as she hit the last step. She looked up at the large, open water and waves. It was like the biggest pool she had ever seen. Her eyes were wide with the look of amazement. I couldn't help but smile with happiness at her wonder.

I have a picture I took that week of her running toward the water, her arms are open wide, as if she is catching the sun in them. Her blonde hair blowing in the wind in her little purple T-shirt and white shorts. It is one of my most favourite pictures in the world. For one of the first times since coming home, she was happy—truly-full-of-joy kind of happy. It was also one of the only pictures we have where she is dry from that week. Keeping that little girl out of the water was a problem. So, we made sure she had her bathing suit on before every walk near the water, and she lived in her puddle jumper for safety. She would sit at the edge of the waves, letting them hit her full-on in the face, and she would laugh with her whole body stimming, her arms and legs wiggling with so much happiness, she could've flown away. And you bet every time we had to leave the beach, she cried big crocodile tears and screamed like we were taking her away from her life force. Her and I are similar that way . . . . Water is just part of your soul, and you can't explain it.

Chase, on the other hand, hated being wet. To him, being wet meant being cold, and he wasn't having it. He was our land baby, and was happiest when warm, dry, and on the blanket on the sand. He would fall asleep under the umbrella in the pile of towels, listening to the waves crash against the shore. We had a place that was safe, where we could all breathe, and we could be a family.

EIGHT:
Seeing Stars

In the fall, we finally had our referrals go through at our local children's treatment centre. They provide occupational therapy, speech therapy, physiotherapy, social work, and some recreational programs and behaviour therapy. For us, it felt like the holy grail of everything we needed for our children to thrive in life. I booked the kids in separately for their assessments. There was no way I was doing two at once.

On the day of Felicia's assessment, I spent the morning trying to memorize her birthday. I kept getting the day and the year switched around, and I didn't want to have to pull out her health card to confirm the information. When you aren't there for your child's birth, you have you learn these details—and my tired brain was having a hard time remembering them.

I followed Felicia like a helicopter around the waiting area as she played with the toys. I couldn't afford for her to run down the massive hallways, I'd never catch her. Within arms' reach was always best. One of the therapists came to get us, and we headed to a small room without windows and with white concrete walls—but it was still bright and cheery. I sat on the carpet with her as we waited. I wasn't really sure what to expect, The lady who had booked us in gave me a brief overview of what would happen, but

I think I assumed one person was doing the overall assessment. Then again, at my level of exhaustion, they could have told me the house was on fire and I would've stood there, processing it.

The occupational therapist entered the room, smiling at us. "We are just waiting for speech, physio, and social work to come in." *Oh, this was a lot more than I was expecting.* "We will get her to do activities and assess her level of competency at each activity. We will talk amongst ourselves, so don't be alarmed by that." I nodded as everyone filed into the room.

The room suddenly felt smaller than it did before. Felicia had zero stranger danger, but my little volcano's temper was in full force that day, and I was already prepared for something to go flying across the room—and I was silently praying she didn't bite someone if they tried to take something from her grasp. They started with basic play, letting her put balls into a tube. They watched her arms and legs and how they coordinated movement between gross motor and fine motor skills. They asked her questions that she paid no attention to trying to assess her speech development. The social worker looked at me and asked to confirm the information on forms. "This is her correct birthday?" *HA! Yes, yes, it is!* I felt proud of myself for remembering. Then, the occupational therapist turned to me.

"What age did she first sit up on her own?" She asked.

"I'm not sure. I don't have that information. She's recently adopted." I shook my head.

"Do you know when she took her first steps or first started eating with a spoon by herself?" She asked as she wrote on her clipboard, and I could feel the blood drain from my face.

"I don't. I could find out from her foster mom and send you that information, though, I'm sure." She nodded.

"Do you have any of these answers?" She handed me a piece of paper. I glanced at the list and shook my head again. I suddenly felt extremely inadequate and flustered.

"I know she was delayed in most skills. She can use a regular cup to drink. We watched her hold a marker in a therapy session we attended, and she's starting to put her clothes on by herself. She's not potty trained yet, if that helps at all." I was grasping for the things I knew she was able to do during the day.

Each therapist had their own set of questions, and I had no helpful answers except for what I had heard in passing during our transition visits and the odd bits I could pick up from the social workers. I was lost. I had missed all her first major milestones. I had no information on them, and I had never thought to ask. I left that assessment feeling like the worst parent in the world. I went home and filed through all our documents, studying each one of them for any thread of helpful information before Chase's appointment.

After surviving the assessments, I knew there would be more of these meetings. More doctors, more therapists. And I never wanted to be caught off guard again. I grabbed a piece of paper and wrote down every answer I knew I could find, so it was accessible. I wrote down doctors' names, addresses, and phone numbers that had followed them in foster care. I wrote down health card numbers and Apgar scores. The more we received, the bigger the binder grew. I kept copies of every document someone might need in labelled tabs, and made copies and easy-to-email PDFs. My three-inch binders proved that my administration background became my biggest strength as a special needs parent. Those binders are my bibles, and—God forbid—if anything happens to me, whoever needs to find the answers would have all the information in one spot.

Chase was picked up first for speech therapy. I had no idea what would be happening in these sessions. He was only still making that annoying grunting sound all the time. He was now two and crawling with confidence. Walking was still a work in progress. I had been wearing him in the baby carrier regularly at home so I could get chores done. He was still only happy if he was touching me. By this point, he hadn't grown much. Twelve-month shirts were just starting to fit—and we were lucky if nine-month pants fit.

We sat in a room similar to the one we had for our assessments—brown carpet, concrete walls, no windows. The speech therapist brought in different toys to try to get him to engage. He loved baby toys that made sounds and lit up. The therapist had a toy gumball machine, big colourful balls were put into the opening at the top, and they would slide down to the bottom. His hand-eye coordination wasn't co-operating, and he would shake with anger when he'd miss the hole. She sat on the floor with him trying to cue baby sounds. She held up a ball. "Ba-ba-ba," she would say to him . . . nothing. He refused to engage with her.

"Sometimes it takes time for them to feel comfortable coming. We will continue to work on basic sounds and mimicking." It wasn't rocket science, but it was help—and I needed guidance on the steps.

I couldn't figure out why Felicia wasn't being picked up as fast as Chase had been. She was three. Services were only covered until children were six years old. I felt like time was ticking. So why didn't she get the spot first? I was told it was important to get them in younger to intervene quickly. But what about her—why wasn't she a priority, when she was struggling just as much as he was? So much time had been wasted already, and we needed help.

Not much time passed before Chase was in full therapy blocks, rotating between speech therapy, occupational therapy, and physiotherapy. We weren't making much progress, but we weren't giving up. Felicia still hadn't gotten the call, but was offered a therapy playgroup once a week. I would take anything I could get for her. She needed social skills—and if a therapist was involved, even better.

The first week of therapy, we were put into a large room filled with toys. There were six other children and their parents. The group was led by three therapists, and parents would stay in the room and help navigate playtime and circle time. Felicia was not playing with any toys appropriately at all at home. I didn't have much hope for this room and its organized toy areas. She could demolish it in seconds if we let her. The therapists tried to engage her in activities like building blocks and the play kitchen, but all she wanted to do was make noise, throw, and then laugh at the chaos she caused. Unless she was in charge of what was happening, it wasn't happening.

One of the therapists showed her a "Cozy Canoe," a blow-up canoe that squeezed her body as it rocked back and forth. At first, there was no way she was being sat in that thing against her will as she tried to squirm out of it, but once it started rocking all went quiet. The therapist started singing "Row, Row, Row Your Boat." We knew she loved movement to the extreme. I mean, this kid would spin for forty-five minutes straight on a spinning chair, stand up, and walk away in a straight line. Her sensory seeking was unlike anything I had ever witnessed. I watched my little, tiny terror go quiet as she rocked, her face calm and content. When the therapist stopped, she looked at her and said, "More." My eyes widened. We needed that at home stat, and I didn't care what it cost!

My goal for these sessions was for us to participate in any way we could. Circle time was the worst. The children would sit in a circle in different therapy chairs, and they would sing, pop bubbles, and take turns picking noisemakers. If someone asked Felicia to participate, she wouldn't. She would scream at them instead. If they wanted her to sit in a chair, she would swipe her hands at them, trying to make contact. She would get up and walk away. I would bring her back, over and over again. If it wasn't on her terms, then it wasn't happening. And she was going to control the show.

Four weeks into the session, I decided that was enough. This kid was going to realize this wasn't an option anymore. She didn't get to run everything. This was the routine, and we were going to participate. I kept my target goal simple: I wanted her to sit with the group for circle. She didn't even have to actively participate, just sit with the other kids. I didn't have Chase, and she had my full attention. I talked to the therapists beforehand, and we agreed she needed to try. I went in determined and sat down on a chair behind her plastic cube chair. We started circle like we did every week, and she went to get up, just as she always had, and I sat her back down instantly. Her eyes flared. I was playing with fire. I knew it and she knew it. She dug her nails into my arm to get a reaction, and I didn't budge. I was learning the different sides of Felicia, and this wasn't autism. This was her need for control—it was her attachment disorder. This wasn't a test of her tolerance for circle time. I was telling her that I wasn't backing down, even when we were in public. I wasn't giving up on her. I was there to stay—and she was going to fight me, tooth and nail. The therapists weren't trained in attachment disorders, so their methods of trying to help in this situation were useless. This situation right there, we had trained twenty-seven hours for in our adoption training. I wasn't backing down. *Game on, kid.*

She screamed in protest. I nodded at the therapists that we were okay. Felicia's body wiggled and swung around at me. I talked to her quietly.

"We are sitting and doing circle. Mommy is sitting with you. You can do this."

She leaned down to bite me. I moved out of the way. She was mad that her teeth didn't land the target, and scraped her nails up my arm instead. I cringed—but if I gave in, it proved she had the upper hand. Her body relaxed for a moment, and she listened to the song they were singing. She clapped her hands, smiling at the therapist. She wasn't stressed . . . she just wasn't getting her way. The song ended, and I must have relaxed just enough to not be paying full attention when her body tensed again. She tried to get up, and I sat her back down, but this time when she let out a scream. She threw her head back at me, making full contact with my face, my glasses digging into the bridge of my nose. When you get hit that hard in the nose by a skull, no matter the size, your eyes instantly water. But I refused to let her go—we were finishing circle no matter what. That blow to the face made me even more determined. It was going to be the battle of the wills to make it to the end. I managed to dodge the next head slam and, when she missed, she tried to bite me again, ending in a scream. She wasn't screaming out of anger—she was doing it just to scream—to make a scene—hoping I would give in. The last song ended, and we did it. We finished circle time. I let her go and let out a happy cheer.

"We did it—you did circle! Now, time to go play again!" She looked at me like, *ugh, finally*, and was gone. I was left battered and bruised, but it was a step we had to take. The parents looked at me without judgement—more of a "we've been there" smile. For the next four weeks, we did our circle time dance of me dodging, protecting her from herself, and walking away with battle scars. But the last week, there were two fresh faces in the room—and at the end of the session, they approached me.

"I'm the principal from the specialized school program we have here. We would like to offer Felicia a spot, starting in January, in our junior kindergarten program. We think she will do well, and we can help her. Would you be interested?" They were seeing that she had potential, just like I did. I looked her, with one eye slightly black from the head butt I had taken earlier in the week.

"Absolutely." With both kids at home, Chase in therapy, and Felicia nowhere near to being accepted yet into the regular therapy program, I needed help. Part of me felt like a complete failure for not being able to have both children at home successfully. All the other parents with toddlers could do it. They loved it. But I didn't have two regular toddlers, and I had to come to terms with the fact I needed help if I was going to be able to keep going. And right now, I was losing my battle—and my arms had all the scars to prove it.

I felt guilty for not having the same connection with my daughter as I did with my son. He demanded everything out of me, but at the end of the day, rocking with him in his room was still my favourite part of the day. He had that baby smell, and he would cuddle in as we rocked and listened to music. I was his person, and he was my little boy. Right from the beginning, I found it hard with Felicia. She did everything she could to fight me. She would pull me in just enough, then put me through the ringer, day after day. Ashley was her person. The moment Ash would come through the door, she would turn into this sweet little girl, asking for love, complete with hugs and kisses. Ashley didn't have the battle scars and the black eyes, or the ringing ears from the hours of screaming—which made it harder for me to explain what was happening during the day. She never saw the full picture, or the intensity this little girl could produce toward another human.

"She's just so . . . hard to love." As the words left my lips, I felt like the worst parent in the world. She had this way of wrapping other people around her finger and pulling them into her world. I was her constant, though. I was the one with her day in and day out, and I was the one who triggered her attachment disorder. *Let me abuse you to see if I can control all that happens around me and to prove that you will leave me, too.* Not too many people can say they have been used as a physical and emotional punching bag by their children, but children with trauma need to know their world is safe. She had lost her birth mom. She had lost her foster mom and siblings. Her world had been turned upside down, and she had no control over any of it—but she could control all her actions, her reactions, and who she let in. And she wasn't about to let me in any time soon.

Ashley had barely been involved with decisions surrounding therapy, Felicia's entrance to school, or the day-to-day struggle. She had thrown herself into work. When she would get home, she would wait until the children were in bed before she came into the house—or, often, she would sit parked down the road in the Jeep, so no one knew she was off work. Her depression was so deep-rooted by this point that she couldn't bring herself to parent, so I made the decisions. What programs we would try, what the therapy schedule would look like, what daycare Chase attended. Therapists, social workers, and daycare teachers all became my community, and an extension to my parenting.

One weekend, we had planned to take the kids to a local park. I wanted to get out as a family, and it was a beautiful fall day. We were barely together, and I was carrying the load of parenting. We woke up and had breakfast, then I dressed the kids and got them ready to go. When I came into the living room, she was sitting in the recliner with a blanket wrapped around her, looking like absolute death.

"We're ready to go." I stood in front of her.

"I'm not going. I don't feel well. I have a migraine." She wouldn't even look at me. *I don't feel well almost every day, but here we are.* I stood staring at her. I felt lost, and she was just gone. My wife, my teammate, the person who had been through everything I had, holding my hand, was not there anymore. I was barely keeping my head above water. I was struggling to keep these kids going, and I didn't feel like I could talk to anyone about it that would truly understand. I knew she was struggling, but I didn't have a lifeline to throw her—I had too many bodies to keep afloat.

"Fine. We are leaving." And I loaded the kids and didn't look back. I was mad, I was heartbroken, I was empty.

We made it to the main entrance to the park and I stopped the truck. I needed to sit for a moment before I got everyone out. It was a perfect fall day, and I was going to try to take pictures of the kids in the fall leaves. The radio was on, the kids loved music so much, and life was always happier if music was playing. I sat looking out at the path and the families walking together, wishing it was *us* all together, happy like that. Then, a little voice piped up in the backseat.

"*Oh, oh, oh, oh . . . Snap back.*" I whipped my head around. Felicia was in her little pink coat, trying to sing along with the radio for the first time. Her little voice trying to keep up to the lyrics. She had never done this before, and I was the only one who was around to witness it. I smiled and laughed through my tear-filled eyes. It wasn't just the song or her singing—it was this glimmer of a little girl I hadn't seen in months, a happy little girl.

I got the kids out of the truck and into the stroller, then we headed into the park. We headed to the grassy hill, covered in leaves. I took them out and tried to snap a few pictures in the fall colours, and then we snapped pictures at the picnic table while we ate a snack, and I texted them to Ashley at home. I think I was just trying to reach her in her depths saying, "Look at what you're missing. You should be here."

Post-adoption depression is not widely talked about, and very much a real thing. The symptoms resemble postpartum depression, and can include anxiety, changes in appetite, fatigue, feeling hopeless, concentration problems, and suicidal thoughts—and can occur in both women and men. It can affect up to 32 percent of adoptive parents, however doctors didn't even start researching further into it until the early 2000s.

For Ashley, it was the darkest place she had ever been—and those days were scary for all of us. She did have anxiety, and felt hopeless to the point of suicidal thoughts. Watching your spouse fade away and feeling like there is nothing you can do is heartbreaking. She was able to get help through counselling, and I am thankful every day that she made that choice—otherwise, she wouldn't be here today.

If you feel like you may have post-adoption depression (PADS), or someone you know may have it, please seek out your nearest professional for help. I will add reading resources and information at the end of this book.

NINE:
Not-So-Magical Holidays

What do you imagine when you think about Christmas with children? The cookie-making, waiting for Santa, the magic in their eyes on Christmas morning?

I have always loved Christmas and everything that goes along with it. I am the kind of person who loves to go to the mall during the Christmas season. I love the energy, the mall decorations—even the crowds. I sit and handwrite my Christmas cards, and wrap every present meticulously with ribbon and bows. My childhood memories are happy and warm, filled with big family gatherings and sitting at the kids table with my cousins. They are the kind of memories you want your children to have.

Leading up to our first Christmas, I tried to stay in the Christmas spirit. The last few years had been hard, as Ashley's family had been grieving her dad, who had passed away suddenly during the Christmas season. I was fine taking on the brunt of the Christmas preparation tasks. I wanted our first Christmas as a family to be as special as we could make it. Ashley's post-adoption depression was still in full swing, she wasn't in a good space, and it was the busy season at work.

I decorated the best I could, with the decorations up high, to keep them out of reach of two grabby toddlers. We were still only living on one level of the house, with the stairs gated off. Ashley had taken Felicia to get the tree at Lowe's. Traditionally, we would go to the tree farm and cut our tree down—but that was asking too much out of everyone this year. We set up the tree in the basement. With the kids not going down there alone, it would be safe.

Trying to find toys and gifts for two children who weren't playing with age-appropriate toys proved to be more difficult than I thought. They didn't have specific interests or favourite shows, which made it hard to search toys stores for something that would be special. They did like stimming over toys that had noise and bright lights, but my ears couldn't take too much more noise in the house. Christmas music was a big hit—especially the songs with odd sounds, like "Jingle Bells."

We would do Christmas at home. We weren't ready to try to go to other people's homes yet. It was just too hard. My parents were away that Christmas at my grandma's house. We would do a different day with them, to spread it out. We asked if Ashley's mom and brother would like to join us after breakfast Christmas day. We planned to take the day as slow and quiet as we could, but we had no idea was what in store.

We didn't know it at the time, but Christmas was what we now call a happy/sad memory for Felicia. Christmas had been a happy time at Melissa's house. They had had a tree with white twinkle lights, from what I've seen from the pictures. They went sledding as a family in the winter, and though she couldn't say it, Felicia held onto these memories tight. It would be the following year when I watched her tiny body sitting in the window as the first snow fell, tears streaming down her chubby little cheeks. She missed her foster family—especially at Christmas. When we helped put up the tree at Ashley's mom's house. Felicia had been excited to help until they turned on the white twinkle lights, then she fell apart and cried again. Ever since then, every Christmas, we always wait for the first snowfall, and hold our breath when the twinkle lights turn on. Some years are easier than others.

Christmas Day, we woke up and made breakfast before we went down for presents. Our goal was to have zero expectations. When Ashley's mom and brother arrived, we all headed downstairs. Felicia was excited about the new ball pit she had gotten from Santa—honestly, we could have probably just gotten that, and the children would've been happy. Chase kept reaching in so he could throw the balls all over the floor. We recently found a video we had taken of this Christmas morning. They were tiny, with little, chubby cheeks. But as we tried to redirect Felicia, she would sass and plunk herself into Grandma's lap. She was in full control mode. We sat and went through stockings and then slowly opened presents. But as soon as the wrapping paper started to tear, Chase stopped coping, and I had to remove him to his room as he began to cry and fuss. While everyone was downstairs, I rocked Chase as he cried and cried. I was hoping I could calm him enough to let him rejoin to finish presents. Finally, I gave in, and put him into his bed. The excitement and sensory input had been too overwhelming, and he slept the rest of the day. After we finished presents, Felicia had her meltdown—and like that, Christmas was over before it had really begun, for both kids. I look back on the videos and pictures from that day and we all look haggard, pushing through for the sake of Christmas.

It wasn't the Christmas I had imagined. It wasn't so magical. It was nothing like the Christmases I had had growing up. Would it ever be?

For children with sensory needs, holidays like Christmas can be very overwhelming—and we learned this the hard way. You add extra visual stimulation with all the bright, loud, and shiny decorations. The sounds of the season, such as music playing everywhere you go. The sounds of family gatherings and people talking. The sounds of paper tearing and family handing them presents to open. The smells of Christmas dinner cooking, baked goods, pies . . . . Now put all these things together, on a child who is already struggling day to day, and it's a recipe for disaster. Imagine turning all your senses on full blast all at once. Now, amplify that with your Christmas experience.

For our children, you can physically watch their bodies stop being able to cope. Felicia's eyes glaze over and become dark. Behaviours escalate, and she needs direct pressure and a quiet room. When Chase was little, he would cry and then just shut down. I would carry headphones and plug them into my phone, blasting The Piano Guys songs so it would drown out the noise while rocking him. We would be in a room full of people, and he would be out cold in my arms, with music filling his ears.

Every year, Ashley and I sit down and review what worked and what didn't. How do we make it more successful next time? Do you take them to gatherings, or does someone stay home? Do we have breakfast before excitement, or let them have the excitement, break for breakfast, then continue afterward if they are doing OK?

There are some years it has taken a week to open Christmas gifts. We let them do Santa on Christmas morning, and the rest gets spread out. We decided that we would do whatever made sense to us, instead of trying to keep up to what was "normal"—and that was hard to come to terms with and explain to some family.

As the children have gotten older, we now struggle with the anticipation holidays. We can normally deflect until a couple days before with things such as birthdays, Easter, and Halloween—but Christmas, it's *everywhere* once November hits. Felicia's excitement and anxiety are in full gear right through until Boxing Day, and then she crashes *hard*. We are now finding the same with Chase as he becomes more aware and more engaged.

As I write this chapter, it is Easter weekend. And this year was a struggle. We have come so far in the last six years. Easter is by far their favourite out of all the holidays. Chase has been running around saying "Happy EEETOR" for about a week, and today, he completely imploded on himself with too much excitement, going down with fiery screams. Felicia's anticipation had kept her up most of the night, and she was up at the crack of dawn and already in little beast mode. She was ready with her sass the moment her feet hit the floor. Add a little bit of sugar and egg hunt excitement to that and *BOOM*—screaming meltdowns all around. Every year we plan, and we aren't sure how it will go, but I am always hopeful next year will be better, and I will try again by altering our plan to let them have this taste of childhood magic.

    I look back at that first Christmas video, we didn't know if the kids would ever understand Christmas. We didn't know if we would ever have family traditions or things that they would like on a Christmas list. We have a greater understanding of what they can manage and what we can handle as parents. I have a better understanding of why people like to go simple during the holidays—it's about the quiet time together versus the big, on-display celebration. This past year, I put up my Christmas village, and the kids liked looking in the tiny village windows. The kids wanted a train around our tree, the same as at Grandma's. I was impressed that they didn't touch it and loved watching it go round and round. Years ago, it would've been thrown. Maybe we will try next year.

    Chase didn't cry in the middle of the field while we got our Christmas tree, like he had done almost every year prior. He took part and had opinions on which one we should get. Felicia liked helping push the cart and watching the guys shake the needles out before wrapping it up. The kids have their own small trees in their room that they can touch and decorate. We don't let them touch our tree ornaments. We tried that one year, and they broke everyone they picked up. We made cookies, and it is an absolute mess every time. I just use throw-away tablecloths now, instead of getting stressed. We do our best to do Sensory Santa instead of fighting the mall lines. Having people who genuinely care and provide such an awesome experience is cherished. A couple years ago, Chase was so excited about seeing Santa, and he got away from me and ran into another family's picture to hug Santa. Special needs families get it, which makes it all more manageable. Everyone had a laugh, and he got an extra candy cane. You change course, you adapt. It won't always be perfect; it won't always go smoothly. But I will try every year to make it special.

TEN:
Bloody Hell

One winter night, I had come home from the barn. It was my place to recharge. I had rescued a neglected pony a few years earlier—she was my escape from the stress of home. I tried to get there as much as I could. As I pulled into the driveway, my phone rang.

"Where are you?" It was Ashley. Her tone was panicked.

"I just pulled in."

"You need to get in here. I think Chase broke his nose." I ran up the steps came through the front door, and Ashley had Chase on the counter. He was crying.

"I can't stop the bleeding."

It took me a bit to register what was going on.

"What happened?" I stripped of my coat and boots and ran up the stairs. She was right—the blood was everywhere. "Where is it coming from?"

Chase started to cry harder because I was home.

"He fell. I think he hit his face on one of the toys on the way down. I had stepped into the back for a minute, I didn't see it . . . ." She looked at me like I was judging her. Chase had just started walking. He had new leg braces, but he was still pretty wobbly on his feet. After being with him all day long every day, I knew how hard it was to take a minute to do anything—let alone try to pee. His face was swelling as I pulled back the ice pack.

"It might be his nose, but it's hard to see. I don't want to chance it. I think we need to go to the emergency room." I couldn't see the source of the blood, though, to even know where to put pressure. Now, if you have children, you know any statement containing "emergency room" is the last thing you want to say—especially with tiny children. But this was beyond my first aid knowledge—and I have a lot of it. I could already see the blood draining from Ashley's face as we spoke. I knew from years of being together that she was not good with blood, and her adrenaline was wearing off.

"You drive us, that way you can stay with Felicia." Chase just wanted me anyway, so I would take him. Our plan made sense as we loaded both children up and drove in the cold, snowy night.

Chase and I headed into triage. I had a washcloth and ice pack soaked in blood as we talked to the nurse at registration. She looked at us sympathetically and gave us an orange popsicle.

"The cold may help," she said as she moved us into the waiting area, and we waited to be called back. Nothing is fast with an emergency room—especially when you have a fussy toddler. I had his diaper bag, which had a few toys in it, in hopes to distract him, but not much worked. His name eventually got called, and we headed to the back to wait some more—but at least we were in a room with a curtain. The nurses gave use wet paper towels to clean up the blood, and they asked their standard questions. I gave them as much as I could as Chase scream-cried in my arms. I hadn't changed my clothes after the barn. I still had my thermals on, and I was sweating and flustered from not being able to calm my poor boy.

The doctor finally came in to see us. I don't know if we had hit him on a bad night or if he was just one of those holier-than-thou guys, but *oh man*, was he a peach.

"What happened?" he asked forcibly as he poked and prodded. "He fell at home while playing. My wife was watching him. I think it's his nose. I can't see where the blood is coming from." Chase screamed and cried to get away from the doctor as he peeled back his swollen lips.

"He just started walking, he's wobbly" I motioned to the AFO leg braces on his tiny legs. "He has special needs."

He glared at me, which caught me off guard. "Where is your wife now? Wasn't she watching him?" His tone was accusatory.

"She's at home with our daughter, and she had turned her back for a minute she didn't fully see what he hit on the way down."

"Does he have a history of any blood disorders?"

"We just adopted the kids six months ago. I don't think so. I'm not sure."

He scoffed at my answer. *Dude, I wish I had the answers, too—trust me.*

"Well, did you check inside his mouth?" he snapped back at me.

No, you asshole—can't you see holding him down for you to look is a two-person job? "No, I didn't think it was his mouth, I thought it was his nose." *Isn't that why we are here—so you can tell me what's going on?*

He shoved his finger into Chase's mouth, and my toddler wailed in pain. "He impacted his front teeth. I will get the nurse to get you the information for the specialist to call in the morning, and a social worker should be by soon."

And with that, he left the room. We sat there as I tried to calm my crying, bloody son. The harder he cried, the more he bled. *Wait—what did he just say? A social worker?*

The nurse finally came back and handed me a paper with the dental surgeon's number on it.

"He can have pain relievers tonight as he needs them. Call here tomorrow" She pointed at the card. "They should get you in pretty fast."

"What about the bleeding?" I looked down at Chase's tear-streaked face.

"It should calm down. Keep him quiet, give him cold things to suck on. It will help. I'll get you guys out of here in a few minutes."

"He said something about a social worker?" I was afraid to ask.

"He doesn't think that an injury this bad could be caused by a fall." I could feel my whole body start to panic and go numb. *What does he think? I upper cut my own kid?!*

"What? We just adopted the kids. You can call my social worker if need be."

She was just the messenger. We were ushered out, and I panic-texted Angela. It was late. I didn't think I would hear back from her until the following day, but she called me right away. She explained that the incident would get sent to Family and Children Services, but she was going to make some calls—and just to pick up the phone when they called the next day. My brain was reeling. We had done everything we needed to make sure he was OK, and this guy was calling a social worker on us? We are the adoptive parents; we are the families the children go to after they've suffered trauma in their lives. I didn't go through hours of interviews and training to end up like this.

It was late by the time we got home. We gave him children's Tylenol at regular intervals and hoped he would fall asleep. His tiny face was double the size and purple from bruising. His bed would need to be changed again in the morning from the bloodstains. I laid in our bed thinking about all of things that could possibly happen after the phone call came. We had spent years trying to build this family, and it only took a few months for us to end up in the emergency room. Maybe we weren't capable of keeping these kids safe. Would the CAS think that as well?

Ashley Biddiscombe

The next day, I waited anxiously for the phone to ring. It finally did that afternoon. The social worker was surprisingly cheerful as she asked me basic questions about what happened. I explained everything in detail, and that we were new parents who had just adopted. I think she heard the panic in my voice.

"Did you have Doctor . . ." She rhymed off his name.

"Yes." To my surprise, she chuckled a little.

"We get a lot of calls when he's on duty. It's OK. You're doing fine. This won't be on your file. Parenting is hard, and I'm sure you're doing a wonderful job. Things like this happen. Don't worry. Take care." She hung up and I let out a breath I didn't know I was holding. She had said the words I had needed to hear.

I never, ever wanted to go through that again. Little did I know, my little Bam-Bam and The Volcano had other plans in store for us over the years. Chase impacted his teeth for a second time, then had to get them removed. Felicia hit her head not once but *twice*, and needed stitches. Both children had various lumps, bumps, bruises, scrapes, and a lot of blood shed. We would soon learn which walk-in clinics were the best and the ones to avoid, who did stitches and who didn't. If I have any parenting advice to give . . . learn first aid before you have kids. It will be the most-used skill you will ever have—and a well-stocked first aid kit is a must.

ELEVEN:
Mother's Day, It's Complicated

"A child born to another woman calls me Mommy. The magnitude of that tragedy and depth of that privilege are not lost on me." —Jody Landers

I thought I was going to be over-the-moon excited for my first Mother's Day. I had been waiting to be able to celebrate for six years. I woke up and felt a kind of melancholy, and it was hard to explain. The only way for me to become "Mommy" was for another woman to lose her children—and in that moment, I wondered how she felt this morning.

We had met the children's birth mom while we had been doing our transition visits. We had the chance to meet her for breakfast one weekend with the help of the children's social worker. Society likes to paint a picture of birth parents in media, making them the villains of the story. So going into this breakfast, we were not sure what we were walking into. You almost want your brain to make them horrible, so it's easier to cope with what is happening. We knew there were some problems from the past, but seeing those things on paper and then in front of you are two different experiences.

We walked into the restaurant and the social worker flagged us over to the table.

"She's just in the bathroom. She's looking forward to meeting you, but she's nervous."

We nodded. So were we.

A young girl in her early twenties came and sat down, her long, dyed reddish hair hung loose, her shoulders curled in, almost as if she was protecting herself. Her face looked exactly like Felicia's, and it almost took me back a little. The faces she made and the way she moved, I had already witnessed in a mini version. We introduced ourselves, made small talk, and ordered our breakfast. She took her time saying what she wanted to say—almost like she was processing as she went. Her sentences were short and trailed off. The social worker helped navigate the conversation. During the meal, she got up and excused herself multiple times. The social explained more about her history. We took note of the things we would have to watch for in our own children as they got older. We weren't there to judge, we were there to learn. We finished our meal and decided we had put enough on her for the day. It was overwhelming. Before we said goodbye, we got a photo of the three of us together—for her and for the kids.

"I'm glad they are going to a loving family. I just want them to be loved."

We reassured her they would be, and that we would send pictures and updates. They would know who she was and that she loved them. While the kids were at Melissa's, she had been able to visit regularly, and now that we were moving them four hundred kilometres away, that would no longer be possible. It was already stipulated that it would be an open adoption—emails and pictures would be shared twice a year, and we would bring the kids up once a year to visit in person. Felicia had a strong connection to birth mom, and she was very much aware of who she was. It can feel like you are doing wrong, even though it's for the right reasons. Moving meant she was going to be gaining her forever family, but it meant losing the constant contact to her birth mom and her foster mom. Adoption isn't as straightforward as it seems, and understanding and respecting the weight of these changes is important.

On Mother's Day, I rolled out of bed, and I felt sad for everyone. The year had been so hard at home. I had poured my blood, sweat, and tears into every day living to make sure we all made it. I deserved Mother's Day. But I had missed the kid's first years. I wasn't there for the NICU with Chase. I wasn't there for first steps and first words for Felicia . . . I didn't carry them for nine months. That woman was six hours away, probably having a hard time knowing that she couldn't even see the kids today. Did she feel like a mom? Did she ignore the day completely, trying to cope? Would she miss the crafty Mother's Day things from school? Was she worrying about how they were doing? Should I have sent her an email?

The first time Chase had a Mother's Day tea at his preschool, I felt like an imposter, sitting there, surrounded by the other moms. I am not sure why—I was doing all the tasks that they were doing every day, but I just didn't feel like I belonged at that table. It was still weird, being called Chase's mommy. It takes time to settle and accept the role as parent, and I was still trying to figure out how to feel that deep connection and love for my kids that birth parents just naturally seem to have for their children. Adopting is like dating—you must learn about each other, earn trust and respect. You have to learn what they like and what they don't like. Love takes time to grow—sometimes, it is not instant. When parents were saying how they missed their children after they went to sleep, I would look at them like they had two heads. I couldn't wait for my kids to go to sleep, and I didn't want to see them until maybe mid-afternoon the next day if I was lucky. Not that I ever left them that long—but a parent can dream about the day their children sleep in. I know now that is also part of burnout—but *hey*, we were struggling pretty bad at that point.

Ashley Biddiscombe

There were times when someone would ask me, "But what about their 'real' mom?" *What does that make me, then—the fill-in?* That narrative fed into my imposter syndrome. I would always answer, "You mean their birth mom?" Her story wasn't mine to tell, and I felt protective over her. She wasn't a bad person, and I wasn't about to portray her that way. People wanted to paint her as a villain, I think, to make themselves feel better. She was still a part of my children; she was an extension of our family, and would be for the rest of our lives. When you adopt, you take on more than just the children—there are sometimes birth parents or birth families. And you are all there to love your children. What child doesn't want more love?

When we had gone through our adoption training, I didn't think I could handle doing an open adoption. I wanted it cleancut. But now, having one, I can't imagine it any other way—and I know now there is no such thing as a clean cut. What you think is best for you isn't always best for your children. Children need to know where they come from. They need to have answers about their own history. Felicia knows her birth mom is her "tummy mommy," and knows that her birth mom couldn't take care of her. She knows that Melissa is her foster mom, and she took care of her until they could find her a forever family, and she is accepting of all that information. I don't think we give children enough credit for what they can comprehend and handle. It may not always be pretty—but it's their story, not mine. My children get to grow up knowing their birth mom is out there and that she loves them, and that's important.

As a mom of children with special needs, there is also an added layer to Mother's Day that many parents don't understand. My children don't even know that the day exists. I have never had them come home excited to give me a homemade gift from school that they didn't have help with, or struggle to make me breakfast in bed on their own. I haven't even had my son say the words "I love you" to me unprompted. I know my children love me, and I don't need a day for them to express that. But when Mother's Day comes around the corner, I never feel like it's "my day." I always think of it a time to celebrate with our parents and grandmothers. Mother's Day is not cut-and-dry in the adoption world or special needs world, so I will leave you with this . . .

To the moms who must live forever,
To those who must make impossible decisions. The ones who sit beside hospital beds and advocate harder and louder than anyone else. The moms who have never had a homemade card, or breakfast in bed. The moms who have never heard their child say "mom" or "I love you." The moms who are managing meltdowns, and are isolated in their homes. Who feel alone in their journey and wonder what motherhood looks like outside of disabilities. To the moms who are living in "the hard." You are the most badass women that have ever lived. Your strength and determination to give your children and your families the best you can doesn't go unnoticed.

Let yourself take a break. Let yourself breathe now and then. Accept the help when it is offered—sometimes, the smallest gifts of kindness will make your life a little brighter. Look at the people who are willing to be your community and—as hard as it can be—ask them for help.

You know your children better than anyone else in this world. Even though they can't always express how they feel, you are their world. The days that are our hardest are always the days they need you the most. You are doing an amazing job, even on your worst day. Being a good mom doesn't mean having the cleanest home. It doesn't mean making cookies and being on the PTA. Being a great mom is showing up, being there when your children need you, and doing what's best for them, no matter what that looks like.

Ashley Biddiscombe

You've got this. And on the days that you don't . . . order pizza, throw on Paw Patrol *for the millionth time, and let chaos reign. Tomorrow is a new day.*

TWELVE:
Isolation

Felicia had started her new junior kindergarten class in January. We would battle to get ready in the mornings. Then the bus would pick her up at the end of our driveway, and she would be gone for half the day to grow and learn with teachers and therapists. Her favourite day was Friday, because she got to swim in the school's therapy pool. With Felicia gone at school, it meant it was just Chase and me during the morning, until the bus dropped her off again at lunch.

As winter turned to spring, life was feeling more manageable with one child at home. I was starting to venture further from home for the first time. We had therapy appointments, but I wanted to do what the other toddler moms were doing—like swimming, children's museums, and playgrounds. We started off exploring parks around town, but with a semi-mobile, sensory-seeking two-year-old, all he wanted to do was sit in the swings. I thought if he had the ability to crawl and explore on his terms, in a safe environment, he would engage more. I wanted him around other children his age, so we headed to a small indoor playground. He would toddle around, throwing toys. He didn't have many play skills, but at least we were in public, throwing someone else's toys. He had come so far, and it was nice to be out with everyone else.

Other moms would often come up to me and ask how old he was. I would respond, "He's two." They'd look at him, puzzled, as they watched him crawl and make baby sounds. I always felt the need to follow up with, "He has special needs." They would give us sympathetic look, and the conversation would end, as they would walked away. I don't know why I felt like I had to disclose that information. I think I preferred the sympathetic look over the judging stares of "why isn't he walking or talking?" I was insecure about my parenting, but at the same time, we were spreading disability awareness among these new moms. Maybe they would think twice about their judgement. Even in a full room of new moms and toddlers, we were still on the outside looking in. I didn't feel like we belonged—our life was therapy appointments, specialists, and social workers. I sat there and watched my son crawl around, and tried to remind myself how far we had come, and not to feel sad for either of us. I didn't let the judgement hold us back. I was determined to be a part of society again, and to feel normal. My son deserved what other kids were experiencing.

I would meet up with friends who had children, and we would catch up. I would sit and watch their children running, talking, and playing as Chase would sit at my feet. I loved their kids as if they were my own, but seeing children the same age as mine thriving and doing age-appropriate things reminded me of how delayed mine were. Our friends could listen, but they couldn't fully understand the level of *hard* I was experiencing at home. I never blamed them for that. They were supporting in the only ways they knew how. I would almost feel more comfortable at the therapy centre, surrounded by therapists, than in our own friend circles. I didn't have to explain myself there. I didn't feel like I had to apologize for my children's behaviour. It was our own little special needs bubble, and stepping out of it was a hard reality, which I had a tough time facing and accepting.

June crept up quickly. Soon, I would have both kids home again full time—but first, I had a meeting with Felicia's school, as part of her end-of-school assessment. The office had called me and said we would be having a "transition to school" meeting. We had already decided that she wasn't ready for the public school system, and neither were we. Jumping into the decision between private school, or full-time therapy was just too hard based on where we were at. I received minimal information about the meeting, but I knew I would be seeing her teacher. I told Ashley I could do the meeting by myself, and I could take Chase, since it was at the therapy centre. We would be fine.

On the day of the meeting, I loaded up the diaper bag with snacks and toys for Chase to play with, and we headed out the door. When we arrived, we were put into a decent-sized meeting room. I tucked Chase on the floor in the corner with his array of things to keep him busy. The door opened, and I was greeted by Felicia's teacher, then the school's speech therapist, occupational therapist, physiotherapist, school liaison, and a few people I didn't know. This was much bigger than I thought, and I suddenly felt overwhelmed. Chase hadn't slept well the night before, and Felicia had been having a hard time at home, and it was a constant fight, followed by a lot of screaming and meltdowns. I was the kind of tired where you feel spacey, and your eyes are swollen and strained, and drinking coffee all day long doesn't make a dent.

We started the meeting, and they went around the room providing updates about their involvement in Felicia's care at school and how she was doing. *I should've told Ashley to come . . . this is a lot.* As I tried to listen intently to everyone speak, Chase noticed I wasn't paying attention to him and he couldn't touch me from where he was sitting. He instantly started to get fussy and noisy. I tried to keep him distracted while half-leaning down, putting balls into a container for him, as I listened to the team talk. But he wasn't happy. This kid wanted my full attention—which, normally, meant me sitting, staring into his soul. I moved him to my lap, where he grabbed at my glasses to throw them on the floor. As I struggled to follow along, we started to get to the transition-out-of-school section of the meeting. They knew she wasn't going to school in the fall, but were able to give me information on other things we could be doing instead, to prepare her for more social interaction.

"So, once she's discharged from the school, she will go back onto the wait list for full therapy services, then?" I asked.

"No, she's discharged from the centre," someone piped in. My eyes snapped up from Chase toward the voice.

"But she still qualifies for two more years of free services until she's six. She's only four." I could feel my confusion and panic sinking in. By this time, Chase was crying, and I was struggling to hold his little, squirmy body on my lap as I tried to offer him Cheerios.

"No, she will be fully discharged from all programs."

"No one told me that when we took this kindergarten spot." My mind was racing. *What will we do? She needs the services. She's not talking in full sentences, she can't draw or colour, she's at the level of a two-year-old.*

And then, the sentence that will stay with me forever . . . .

"You should have been a better advocate for your daughter."

The speech therapist glared at me from the far end of the table. *What did she just say?* The whole room went silent as I sat there, stunned. I could feel the heat rising in my face and my body starting to tingle from embarrassment. We had spent the last six years advocating for ourselves and for children we didn't even know existed. We advocated for ourselves so we could adopt these children. We advocated to see specialists and to get into this therapy centre. But I had to be a better advocate for my daughter?

Someone awkwardly tried to move on. In that moment, in a room full of people who knew my children were adopted, not one person said a word to stand up for us. Not one person defended our journey. I couldn't find the words. For the first time ever, I felt completely isolated in a world that was supposed to be filled with the support of professionals who understood. It was supposed to be our safe bubble away from the outside world. I can't remember what happened after that. All I remember is packing up Chase, and crying all the way home. I had never felt so alone, and had no idea what we were going to do going forward.

Once I got myself together, which I will admit took a few days, I decided that under no circumstance was I ever going to let anyone make me feel less-than again. You want a better advocate, *game on*.

To this day Ashley calls it my "mama bear side." It comes out in full force now and then, and I will admit, sometimes, I am a little scary. But I look at her and tell her no one else will advocate for our children except for us, and I refuse to let them fall through the cracks of another system. The only people who get things done in the special needs world are the ones who are louder, and know the ins and outs.

As Chase moved through the centre's therapies, I started noticing things that weren't parent-friendly, and definitely not geared toward adoptive families and children with trauma. Like many things in the public sector, there were holes—and plenty of opportunities to fall through the cracks. Chase was aging out of the therapy centre, and I was feeling increasingly driven to make change—not only for my own children, but for other families like mine. We were offered a parent survey during our exit meeting, and I gladly accepted the opportunity. When I realized that this might be my chance to be heard and maybe be able to change what was happening, I filled it out and added three extra pages about our experiences and where I thought the centre needed change. I told them about our meeting, and what was said to me, and how I felt. I told them about the lack of trauma training and how that was important. I spoke about how the constant change in speech therapists hindered my son's progression. I didn't hold anything back, and I even included ways these problems could be simply solved. My parent survey was escalated to three different departments, and I had multiple phone conversations with staff. I was told no one had ever been so honest, or had had real, plausible solutions that could be used before. I finally felt like I was being fully heard by someone who wanted things to change, too.

Recently, I was approached by one of the women who I had interviewed with, and was informed that all staff will be going through trauma training and learning about the effects of trauma on childhood development because of my survey. I am proud to say I was part of that change. It was our family that helped make that happen.

Change never happens on the sidelines, so when a spot opened on the board of directors for the centre, I put my name in, and got it. I am not a vindictive person by any means, but thinking about the look on that speech therapist's face in that meeting makes me laugh, because now, I'm technically in a group that helps make the higher-level decisions.... *Joke's now on you... I'll show you what an advocate does.* An advocate it stands up for all families like mine, to make sure *that* conversation never happens again, and that no one feels isolated in a place that they are supposed to feel safe.

"The wheel that squeaks the loudest is the one who gets the grease." —Josh Billings

THIRTEEN:
Getting Answers

Looking back, I think I took 2017 for granted. At the time, I would've told you that was insane. I was tired and stressed, searching desperately for answers about what our future looked like. We were finally getting our feet under us again, and what we had in place was perfect for both kids. Even though we were still fighting for services for Felicia, we decided to try a Montessori school that focused on hands-on learning, self-care, and independence. The school was able to bring in one-on-one support, and Felicia was loving every moment. Transitions were still hard for her, especially at drop-off, when I would hand her over to her teachers—but slowly, she was learning the routine.

One morning at drop-off, we were standing by the coat racks at the school and, unprovoked, she hugged me goodbye. It was the first time she had shown me any sort of physical love. She had hugged and kissed Ashley from the moment they met, but she had never done it with me before. I stood there, shocked, taking in the moment, as I watched her skip into the classroom. She was thriving and learning, and I was relieved.

In the fall, I went as her support on her first school field trip to the pumpkin patch. I was excited to be doing it, just like all the other parents. We walked through a corn maze, rode on a hayride, and got to pick a pumpkin to bring home. Of course, she wanted the largest one she could find. We settled on a medium one and a gourd.

This year, we would be trying out trick-or-treating for the first time. The children's centre was holding an indoor event, which was perfect. The children could be in their costumes in a place they felt safe, and I didn't have to worry about Felicia trying to walk into people's homes or Chase struggling going up house's front steps. If either child had a meltdown, we would be surrounded by support and other parents who understood. Chase was dressed up as The Hulk and Felicia was Spider-Man. Her costume even had built-in muscles, which she loved. Ashley painted both of their faces, and off we went. The kids did amazing. It was a successful outing, and we were so proud of them.

Fall turned into winter and, as we approached Christmas, a letter was sent home with Felicia that said she needed a top hat, scarf, and white shirt for the school concert. I was nervous. She was holding it together at school, but on the stage, in front of a room full of people—that seemed like a huge stretch.

On the night of the concert, we sat in the audience with all the other parents and watched our kids on stage, dressed up as little snowmen. The large room was full of parents and family, and I took note of how visually overstimulating and loud it was. They started the music, and I winced, waiting for her to move. To my surprise, nothing happened. She was up there with her peers, trying to sing along and do the hand actions, and for the first time ever, I felt hopeful that she would succeed. All the hard work, screaming, biting, and hitting led to this moment. We were at our child's Christmas concert. This was a moment I had always wanted as a parent.

Chase had hit the resource jackpot. We had started him in preschool a couple mornings a week. The mornings that the kids were at their programs, I had freedom for the first time in over a year. I was able to get shopping done without the struggle of meltdowns and car seats. I would stop and get a coffee, and drink it while it was still hot. I would head out to the barn and brush my horse, and I felt like I could breathe. All the small things I took for granted before bringing the kids home were now small luxuries I held onto very dearly twice a week. Eventually, I would go on to join the preschool's volunteer board of directors, I was able to put my work skills to use, and felt like I was contributing back to the program that gave me so much sanity during the week.

We were waist-deep in occupational therapy, speech therapy, and physio. Our calendar was a rainbow of appointments, filled to the brim. Chase's therapy team was solid and was making huge strides in his gross motor skills—which, for him, meant the start of independence. We worked on balance while he walked, safety going up and down stairs, eating with a spoon, and playing with toys. Speech therapy, however, was a different story. He had multiple speech therapists in a short period of time. The turnover was high, and every time a new one would come through the door, they would have to start from the beginning. Because of Chase's adoption trauma, he didn't trust new people. You had to work hard for that relationship, according to him. He threw toys at them, refused to participate, screamed, and rolled on the floor. Clearly, their free play methods weren't going to work—so I asked if I could make suggestions.

He would work hard for me, so I brought in his booster seat from home and sat him down in front of me, the same way we did at our dining-room table. I took over as lead therapist in speech. Our actual speech therapist would sit behind me, telling me what to do, and I would execute. It wasn't ideal, but it worked. They kept trying to bring in behaviour therapists, and they would run through suggestions for each behaviour he had. I would sit and tell them that it wasn't behaviour-related but adoption-related. Over and over, I would say, "No, that won't work because . . . ." I was frustrated. I knew him inside and out. It wasn't behavioural, it was attachment. You can't keep changing therapists and expect him to cooperate. We had a team meeting, and we had Angela call in to explain childhood trauma and how it related to Chase. Ashley and I sat there, letting her do her thing, as we watched light bulbs start to go off in our team's head. They got it, finally. We came up with a solid plan for his occupational therapist to join his speech sessions. He trusted her, so she could take over my spot, and I could sit and watch as they would slowly work on relationship-building through activities and play.

I always found that the adoption and special needs worlds work parallel to one another, but rarely cross lines into each other's specialities. It was becoming clear the lack of information that the therapists had about the effects of childhood trauma and how it was affecting their therapy sessions with Chase. I always joked with the therapists, "My kids will push your education and training to the brink." And it was true. Chase was forcing them to look for more creative and personal ways to help him in therapy. I think my kids teach people more than they get taught themselves sometimes. They force people to look beyond the textbooks and what they've been taught to find other solutions, and we were about to see that again in our upcoming appointments.

We were noticing in therapy that Chase's left side was weaker than his right. We questioned the possibility of cerebral palsy. He had been referred to a neurologist, and we were waiting on a date for his MRI. At the same time, we were also starting the process of getting a psychological assessment done for Felicia. I was pushing for the diagnosis of autism. I knew diagnosing girls was harder. Every doctor we came across up until then had said, "No, I don't think it is autism. She's too social, and she makes eye contact." It was like her intense sensory-seeking meltdowns and delays were not important, and social and eye contact was their deciding factor. *Seriously*? In my gut, I knew, and I wanted the right professional, who knew girls on the spectrum. In our world, getting a diagnosis meant help. It meant resources and funding. Without that piece of paper, we were stuck.

Around all this happening, Ashley was coming out of her post-adoption depression depths and fog, and was wanting to be actively involved in parenting again. For the last year and a half, I had manned the ship, keeping everyone afloat. I won't lie—I resented her for it for a long time, and it wasn't easy to pull that nail out of the marriage coffin. I had everything tied together right then, with the flimsiest string in a shabby, little bow. It was all working, and I was terrified of letting go and letting her hold the strings, too. What if she let go again? What if all of this unraveled? What if I unraveled? She really had no idea what I was going through. I was breaking some days. Did she even see it? Then again, I wasn't telling her, either. Letting her in to actively help me parent was not easy, but there was a glimmer of my wife and my teammate, and I desperately needed her to help take the load.

Chase's MRI was finally booked. Felicia was headed to spend the day with Nana and Papa, which would be much more fun than a hospital. Chase was going to have to be anaesthetized. The MRI was forty-five minutes, and there was no way you could expect a child to lay still in a huge, noisy machine. Paediatric MRIs had to be done at the children's hospital, which was about an hour and a half away, so it would be an all-day event. After our earlier stint in isolation with Chase, this didn't seem too bad.

We arrived and walked through the maze of hallways to the MRI department. One parent was allowed back, and I knew how he reacted to nurses and doctors, so I stayed with him. He laid on the bed in his tiny hospital gown, unsure of his surroundings, and the mask went on his face. His little body panicked, and I talked to him as I held him tight like a burrito in the blanket, telling him he was safe. He was out cold in five seconds. My strength is procedures with the kids. When a doctor asks, "Are you OK? Do you want me to get a nurse to hold him?", I honestly feel pretty solid and calm. I can only imagine how many parents don't, though. The hardest part for me, though, is walking away and worrying we won't make it back in time for when they wake up. My kids have been through enough loss and fear. We need to be there for when they wake up, and to know we didn't leave them. We always have time to go for coffee and get a bite to eat during these tests, and I constantly worry, checking my phone, to make sure we have time to walk back. Ashley shakes her head at me and laughs. I can't help it.

The MRI was done, and we went to get him from recovery. We had watched the other parents take out their sleeping children earlier, so we were expecting a groggy little boy. But when we came around that corner, our blonde little boy was sitting up eating a popsicle. The recovery nurse was with him.

"He was the fastest wake-up I've ever seen." Leave it to our kid to leave his mark. Once we got him to the Jeep, our happy little boy turned, and the happiness was gone, and he raged. He screamed and cried the full hour-and-a-half drive home. As he clawed at his car seat harness, all I could think was *sleepy little angel, my ass* . . . our kid was tripping hard, and in the moment, I was thankful for how little he was.

Results came a few weeks later, and we found ourselves in the neurologist's office, waiting. I had no idea what to expect. The neurologist opened his file as we sat across from him.

"He doesn't have cerebral palsy."

Shit, I was convinced that was it . . . .

"He does have an underdeveloped cerebellum, though—which is at the base of his brain."

I did well in high school biology, but I was going to have to listen closely to this to understand.

"It's bilateral cerebellar hypoplasia."

That's a lot of words together.

Only the Strong Survive

"The cerebellum is in charge of filtering information from the brain to his muscles, and if that is underdeveloped, the messages cannot pass properly—which explains his motor and speech delays, wide-leg walking, and balance issues. He's also at risk for seizures. We will have to repeat MRIs regularly to watch it, to make sure it's not progressive."

"Progressive how?" I asked.

"In some cases of cerebellar hypoplasia, the cerebellum can continue to deteriorate and shrink in size. Best-case scenario is that it's not that kind, and it stays stable. Do you have any questions?" I had all the questions . . . . Would he talk, climb, potty-train? Would he be independent? I will admit I was scared and confused. What I didn't know in that first meeting was that this is the first time the neurologist had ever seen this in person. Cerebellar hypoplasia is rare in humans. It's more often seen in animals. I am a research junkie, and I needed to know more, but there wasn't any information to be found. So, I turned to where I knew other parents were—other parents are filled with random information. I searched "cerebellar hypoplasia" on Facebook and, *what do you know, there was a group*! The group was small—only around a thousand parents from all over the world were in it. This was rare, but as I scrolled through posts and videos, I saw little humans just like mine, with the same wide stance, wobbly walk, wearing glasses, using walkers and leg bracing . . . . The future was unknown, but we had answers—not all the answers, but it was a start. For now, our goal was progression whatever that may be and life skills that could make him as independent as possible.

In the winter, we started having more behavioural issues with Felicia at school. At pick-up, the "how was the day" conversation was getting more concerning and we were having more bad days than good. Her one-on-one support worker had left for a new job, and they were trying out someone new—and they had added new students into the class, who hadn't been transitioning well. Felicia's little world had been turned upside down yet again. We threw as many coping resources at the school as we could to get her through the mornings. We added extra sensory breaks, noise-cancelling headphones, compression vests, chewelry—anything we could think of that may help keep her calm. We were about to start her psychological assessment, and hoped to get some answers.

Ashley and I sat down and filled out a stack of questionnaires which would be followed by meetings at the psychologist's office, and she would also observe Felicia in the classroom environment. We felt confident in her and the plan. Weeks later, we sat in her office for the report review.

"First, I want to say she is a wonderful little girl—and don't forget at as we go through all of this in the next hour. There's a lot."

We nodded. *Give it to us, straight doc.* And then she did.

"She has the most intense sensory-seeking behaviours I have ever seen in my career...."

And the next hour, we had all our suspicions confirmed—and then some. The report was so much more thorough than I was expecting—but this was the document that would be our "go-to" for years to come. As we left the office, I felt relieved—but also a wave a sadness that I hadn't been expecting. There is something about seeing your child on paper that makes it all a reality. You move through your day-to-day life knowing where your child is in development, but these documents, remind you of all the hurdles you have yet to face, and the uphill climb your child has. We didn't just leave with the diagnosis of autism, but also intellectual disability under the first percentile—meaning out of one hundred people, her intellect was at the lowest end of the spectrum. She also was diagnosed with attachment insecurities, and she was suspected of having ADHD. All of this would be piled on top the genetic abnormality that we were still waiting to figure out with the geneticist. Five different labels now sat on Felicia's head. It was a heavy diagnosis for such a little girl. But this document had to help us—this tiny human had fallen through so many cracks in her life already.

As winter turned into spring, the calls from the school started coming more regularly, and I was picking her up at least once a week early due to aggression toward teachers, eloping through the school halls, and erratic behaviour in the bathrooms. And her need for control took over. I have to give this Montessori school credit—they tried their absolute best—but at the end of the day, they were a regular school for typically functioning children, and did not have the special needs background or supports. Every teacher and the principal wanted to see Felicia succeed. She didn't want to be picked up early, and the aggression toward me trying to get her into the truck was escalating to a scary level. I didn't know how much longer we could hold on, and I was praying it would just all stop and we could go back to when she was hugging me at the coat racks. I couldn't get anything done while she was at school, in fear that the phone would ring. When she escalated, I was the only one who could take her on. I often had Chase with me during pick-up, and keeping us all safe was my goal.

During one pick-up, I was waiting outside, with Chase in my arms, and she came out of the school like a tornado, which caught me off guard. I didn't get a call that day, so I was expecting her usual smile as she skipped out the door—but not today. Intense screaming filled the air, and she was trying to claw her way back into the school, trying to get away from her teacher. I caught her by the hand while balancing Chase on my hip. She thrashed and swung her body around. *We just need to make it to the truck—just get us to the truck.* There were a couple other parents at midday pick-up, and I tried to keep my head down and focused on my daughter and not the stares. I was somewhat used to the stares. I had carried this kid out of more places in full meltdown mode than I could count at this point. But it was different among strangers, versus those I'd have to see every day at pick-up.

Then, in a blink of an eye, she was lying in a puddle on the asphalt while she tried very hard to aim her tiny feet at my legs, wanting so desperately to make contact with my shins. One of the other moms cautiously approached our chaos.

"Let me take him to the truck for you."

And I handed Chase over, nodding. That tiny gift of compassion helped me find the strength in that moment to keep going. In a swift motion I picked Felicia up out of the puddle in a way that would protect both of us—the best way I could—and made it to the truck. We were now both soaking wet in muddy water as she thrashed around. If you watched a video of someone trying to tackle an alligator, I'm sure it would look the exact same.

As she started to get bigger and heavier, I always feared the day I wouldn't be able get her out safely—but we were still at a point where when I needed to, I always found the strength to hoist her up and lift her into her car seat. These episodes would exhaust me, though, later—the kind of exhaustion that comes from your core. Most days, I could crank the music up loud and it would snap her out of her screaming, and she would calm down on the car ride home, but lately, that wasn't happening. I was sure that her ear-piercing scream could be heard from miles away. We got home, and I put Chase in his crib, where he would be safe while I cleaned Felicia up, as her meltdown continued. She needed to be kept safe, and I needed to breathe—but that wasn't going to happen anytime soon. She screamed for the next four hours without stopping. By the end, she had popped all the blood vessels around her eyes, leaving little pock marks, like a raccoon. She scratched her skin and mine, and when she finally stopped, her vocal cords were hoarse. She fell asleep in her bed, and I cried silently in the bathroom. We couldn't keep living like this.

Only the Strong Survive

April was my breaking point. These long, intense meltdowns were happening multiple times a week. One morning, the phone rang, and my head dropped . . . it was the school. The principal had her in her office yet again, and things had escalated. She had hit one of the teachers and run out of the classroom. They had moved her to the principal's office to try to calm her down. She had picked up the principal's fresh coffee and promptly whipped it across the room, somehow missing anything important. When that didn't satisfy her rage, she grabbed her laptop and it made full contact with the wall. When I arrived at the school and opened the door, she was sitting, playing with post-it notes on the principal's desk. I took her hand and quietly walked her out the door and to the truck. I was at a loss for words, a loss for answers, and a loss for hope.

We took a few days at home. I was trying hard to dig deep and find compassion for this little girl, who was no longer coping with any aspect of life. *You had one job, kid—you just had to go to school.* But it wasn't just school. It was testing her every threshold, and she couldn't be stretched any further. At home, she was quieter as she decompressed. She tried hard to get my attention in positive ways, but I was just so worn down, I didn't have much left to give her in return. She wanted to learn, but couldn't handle the school environment. Could I do this at home? Did I have a choice? School was no longer safe, the teachers weren't safe, and she wasn't safe from herself. I picked up the phone and called the principal. I was done fighting, and we were done with school.

FOURTEEN:
You Do What You Gotta Do

How was I going to juggle Chase's therapy, preschool, and activities, and homeschooling Felicia? Luckily, Ashley's mom and my parents lived close by, and were willing to be the drop-off zone as I played taxi. We had also been referred to a young woman who was a respite worker and was willing to come take Felicia for a few hours a week. Respite workers are saviours. To have an extra set of hands to help keep your children safe and occupied does wonders for your mental health. It was going to be about making our own community—which was easier said than done.

Homeschooling gave us mass amounts of freedom to come and go as we pleased. I was no longer tied to school pick-ups and drop-offs, or the risk of the phone ringing. We did day trips, parks, children's museums, indoor playgrounds, anything to keep the kids busy when we weren't on the run with therapy. It also gave us the opportunity to research programs that ran during the day. We weren't pressed to sign up for recreational programs on evenings and weekends, so I focused on daytime options. They were the quietest—which was perfect for two children who struggled with loud environments. I got braver, taking two children to the grocery store alone. It wasn't easy, but I refused to be stuck in the house under house arrest any longer. I could do this. We just had to try.

Once summer arrived, all programs and therapies had stopped, and we were on our own to keep busy. Becca, our new respite worker, was ready to try a summer day camp that the therapy centre was holding with Felicia, so off I sent them for a week to try it out. Becca was my eyes, ears, and creative brain at camp. Felicia was in safe hands, and there was swimming. If Felicia was in the water, she was happy. It also gave me a chance to have one-on-one with Chase, which we hadn't had in a while. We explored trails at the conservation area, went to splash pads and parks, and took our family vacation. Summer felt like a well-deserved break. When Felicia and Becca weren't at camp, Becca was taking Felicia on outings—and even riding the city bus without fear. She was willing to try things that I couldn't, and it got Felicia into the community in new, fun ways. People come into your lives at times when you need them most—and *man*, did I need her.

I knew we weren't sending Felicia back to school come September. I had a lot of PTSD to work through after our exit from Montessori, and she was still struggling with regulating herself. There weren't any options we felt confident in, so we decided not to rush anything. I started to book the kids into special-needs-geared programs—such as swimming, art classes, gymnastics—and Chase still had preschool. Our goal was to get out into the community safely while gaining social and group skills.

Around this time, we lost a good friend to cystic fibrosis. She was only thirty-four. Mary was the perfect mix of cynical and realistic. You could talk to her about almost anything. She spent her life knowing everyday was a gift, and to live for the small things, like the simple joys of sprinkles on a cupcake or enjoying the perfect song. When she became a parent, we watched her pour herself into parenting, like she was soaking up every moment she could. When her daughter came out as transgender, I watched a parent fully embrace their child as who they were—no questions asked. And then, I was one of the fortunate people to watch a fierce advocate emerge. She stopped at nothing to bring education and acceptance to the school board—and anyone who would listen—in hopes of creating a more aware and accepting world for her child.

The last time I saw her, she was standing in our front hall. She had brought over craft supplies for Felicia and Chase. Her breathing and coughing were getting worse, which meant the scar tissue in her lungs had built up after years of fighting infections. She was on oxygen all the time then. She had just finished going through the process of finding her daughter the perfect adoptive home. She wanted to make sure that her child was settled and safe before her health declined further. Mary gave up everything for her daughter—to make sure she would be happy and safe—and fought until the very end. Her last message to me was a Glennon Doyle post on Facebook about how, as parents, we are good and normal—and it is our children that make us crazy. I look at this post now and then. Mary knew that I would need the reminder and the laugh. We always knew we wouldn't have her forever—but you are never fully prepared for when the time comes to lose someone. When she passed away, I vowed that if she could be that strong, and fight that hard for her child while being so sick, then there was no reason we couldn't do the same. I know I wouldn't be the parent and advocate I am today if hadn't been for Mary. She left an impact on our lives like no one else.

As we immersed ourselves in specialized programs, I found myself sitting in waiting rooms with other parents. Some, I knew from teaching years earlier, and some were just like me, struggling to find services—navigating a world that wasn't quite made for our children. We would talk about the happy, and dance around the hard and sad—without fully letting ourselves go there. My kids were often in the junior classes, and the older children in the later classes. I found myself watching the parents of the older children, fascinated by the ease that they moved with. I felt like a ball of stress, waiting for every meltdown, stressed that time was passing and we were missing target years for therapy. They sat and talked about their kids, and they just seemed to be at a different level—and had this essence of comfort about them. *I want to look like that. How do I get there? Will I ever be like them?*

If another parent turns to you and says, "It will get better," you can't even fathom what that means. When you are in "the hard" and they don't know *your* hard, how could they even say that to you? "The hard" is the beginning of your children's diagnosis, or when something changes in your child's diagnosis—when you are struggling to find your place in the world. You are struggling to find coping strategies for everyone, and your whole world feels upside down. You are drowning in the what ifs—the grief of what could have been still lingers, just out of reach. You don't have a community and you aren't quite sure how to find one. It's like you are on your own little island, watching all the boats go by. You are screaming and waving, and no one seems to be waving back.

What I didn't know at the time was that those parents of the older children who seemed so at ease were at a level of acceptance, and the only way to achieve that was get through "the hard" and let yourself grieve all of it. Acceptance is not giving up on advocacy or the future—it's accepting that your child is who they are, and that your life does look different, but that different isn't bad. I can look back now and realize this is something Mary had learned. She had known the secret well before we did. I think she learned it growing up as a child with a chronic illness. It made her wise beyond her years. Maybe I should have listened a little closer.

Acceptance is allowing yourself to look at your child and say, "quality of life comes before anything." To the point of acceptance that your child may never verbally speak, but changing your goals to any form of communication. Maybe your child will never live on their own. But how do we teach life skills to get them as far as we can? How can we provide the best possible life for our children? The parents who were sitting across from me already knew this secret, and it would take me years to learn and even touch the edge of it.

We started growing our community slowly, and I realized what I provided to so many families as an instructor for so many years. As I sat in those waiting rooms, I was able to pick up a book for the first time in two years and polish off a couple chapters while my children made great creations in art class and burned out their energy in swimming. I went from the stress of waiting for calls from the school to enjoying watching my kids succeed in programs, their smiling faces coming out to the waiting room, showing off their creations, or the "mommy, did you see me jump off the side of the pool?" conversations on the way home.

Before I move on with the rest of this story, I want to make sure I take the time I say thank you to everyone who has been in our lives, who has watched my children grow and gain skills I never thought they would achieve.

To the coaches, instructors, support workers in our lives,

As a coach, you can get lost in the work sometimes, and not fully realize the impact you have on families that you see each week. I know how hard you work. I was an instructor for therapeutic horseback riding for almost twelve years. I miss it every day, and I would go back in a heartbeat. I saw hundreds of kids and adults come through our doors. I know how you agonize about lesson plans and how to keep the children engaged week to week.

I met some of the most amazing parents in the world—and now, as a parent myself, I see them differently, with even more respect.

Some riders came with support workers, some parents would stay and watch, others would head out for a coffee. At the time,

I didn't fully understand the ones who left. Why wouldn't they want to stay and watch their children? *I would ask myself.* Today, I know that coffee was so much more.

For some parents, you are one of the few adult interactions a parent gets to have in a week. We are so excited to see another adult, I think we implode sometimes. Sometimes, we toss our kids at you and run back to the car, because that time alone is so precious.

My kids were in half-day camp for one day recently. I know what you're thinking . . . half-day, no big deal. I'm telling you . . . two and a half hours to myself . . . alone . . . biggest treat of my life. Take all of my money for all the half-day camps!

I got a coffee, and I walked the aisles of a bookstore for the first time in years. It was the first time in months I felt like I could breathe. I felt like an old version of myself for a moment in time. I knew my kids were safe and taken care of. Even if they were causing a massive hurricane at gymnastics, they would be OK.

Reality is, I can't take my kids to many stores—between the sensory overload, and my son who is a runner, and doesn't wait it isn't easy. As they get bigger, containment is harder. I avoid taking them at all costs on errands, and if I have to, it's a get-in-and-get-out situation. My daughter is a bit better now that's she's older, but Chatty Cathy will go up to anyone and talk away. She touches everything, she bumps into everything. It's always a high-alert situation. So, those two and a half hours were precious . . . the kind where the store isn't open until ten, but you sit in your car with a hot *coffee*, with your music on or in silence, and wait for the store to open, kind of precious.

What coaches and support workers don't realize is that it's more than the sport or respite care. It's creating independence for our children—a space that they can safely belong in the world. A space made just for them.

Ashley Biddiscombe

For parents, it's peace of mind. It's an hour where our kids our happy and we can have that coffee—have that break and recharge. It's time where you stop worrying about the future or that test result from the children's hospital. It's not a specialist appointment or managing the meltdown or being knee-deep in school IEPs. We sit and watch our children succeed—and sometimes, that's what keeps us fighting for more.

What you provide for families goes beyond your four walls, and if you are ever questioning why you do what you do . . . I'm here to tell you, it matters more than you'll ever realize.

—This Special Needs Mama

FIFTEEN:
When the Baby Door Closes

Whether you are ending your fertility treatment journey, deciding not to have any more children, or can't have any more children, you must face the "baby door" closing.

In 2018, we found out that the birth mom was pregnant again, which we weren't completely surprised about. But we were also thinking we had more time before we had to have "the talk" about where we sat on the subject.

When a birth mom who has already had children apprehended gets pregnant, CAS steps in to assess their ability to create a stable home for the child, even if their children have already been have been adopted. The goal of the CAS is to provide support to birth parents and try to keep families together, if possible. All parents make mistakes. Saying that a child can't stay with a birth parent—if they have shown they have been able to get their life together and make better life choices—would be unfair to both the parent and the child. In the easiest way to explain it all obviously, with many variations and considerations: if the birth parents have not been able to turn things around and the child is at risk of going into the foster care system, then next of kin is looked at for potential custody—then finally, the adoptive parents of any siblings, in hopes to keep them together.

On our end, we tried to stay realistic about our odds of being contacted. However, we still had to be prepared for the possibility, and try not to get excited by the idea that we could have the chance to have a baby. This baby would be our children's half-sibling. The likelihood this child also having challenges was high, but we already had every specialist on earth in our roster. We knew the system and our resources. I would've rather navigated specialists than try to add another foster or adoptive family into our mix to keep track of. We were of the mindset of *what's one more?* What if we got this baby right away, and we could get on top of all the assessments sooner—and if there were problems then we already knew, early intervention was the key.

Baby three arrived, and the system stepped in, as predicted, and we held our breath. A few months later, I received an email from the birth mom, proudly stating that CAS had closed her file and she was able to parent him. I was floored. We were worried for her and for him. They were still our children's blood relatives, and we wanted to see her thrive. There was nothing we could do, so we checked in now and then with our update emails and hoped for pictures. His resemblance to Felicia is uncanny. There are zero questions that he is her brother.

Just when you think you have your emotions under control . . . *bam*, that tempting little-baby possibility, dangling just out of reach, makes itself known again.

"But you've got your kids. Isn't that enough?" you may be asking.

Yes, we do, and we love them profusely—but there is something about that missed time in the early months that always eats at me.

My son was nineteen months old when he came home. Very delayed and very small, he was only the size of a nine-month-old. He was still on a formula bottle and just crawling. You could argue I got my baby stage. But we missed the first milestones, and it was hard not to feel guilty that we hadn't been there. Not that we had any control over that at all—it's just the thought, *what if we had found them sooner?* What if I had been there when he was in the NICU—could we have avoided the separation anxiety? Could I have been in a position to fight for services sooner, and gotten ahead? Playing these games with myself gets me nowhere, so I settle on the fact we all just weren't ready for each other then, and move on.

As Chase grew, I had a tough time letting go of the small things. But for me, they were big things. As he grew, he didn't rock with me as much before bed. We were saying goodbye to the nighttime bottle, and he was starting to feed himself. We were still knee-deep in diapers, but I felt like I had gotten this small taste of what having my baby was like, and then *poof*, he was a toddler, as he should have been all along. But that grieving part of me wanted to hang on just a little while longer. Ashley was the one pushing him to use a cup and trying to get him to walk. I wasn't ready to say goodbye to the baby yet.

We did have the "baby talk" again over the years. Ashley wanted to make sure I was one-hundred-percent sure I didn't want to try one more IUI, like the doctor had suggested. I had ended that chapter abruptly, and she wanted to make sure I wasn't going to have any regrets. In 2019, a letter came in the mail from the fertility clinic. It was a "what do you want to do with the donor sperm that was frozen" letter. We had three choices: pay the storage fee for another year, dispose of it, or donate it to science. Could you imagine taking hormones and parenting two children with special needs? I surely could not. I knew my limits, and that was beyond them. I knew in my gut I didn't want to go back to the clinic ever again. I was done. However, something about signing that paper hit me like a wall. It was the final goodbye. We couldn't afford the storage fee for another year for it to sit there. The thought of someone pouring five thousand dollars of our money down the drain literally seemed insanely wasteful, and there was no money-back guarantee on these things. So, I checked off "donate to science." Maybe someone would learn something valuable from our misfortune—something that would help someone else. I sealed up the envelope and put it in the mail, crying over six vials of sperm we would never use. I was officially done, and a wave of infertility grief hit me again.

We plugged through, and I was feeling good about our little family. The baby stuff we had used was boxed up and put away into storage. I wasn't ready to face getting rid of it all quite yet. There is something so final about giving away baby stuff, which I think everyone goes through. The "baby door" was closing again, but we were the ones saying it was OK—we had control with this choice. Ashley agreed to do it slowly. I only kept the outfits that our children wore on the first day we met them, and their first pairs of shoes—and I have almost all of Chase's old leg bracing. Not that I want to do all-nighters and diapers with a screaming baby—hell, I'm still doing that with our seven-year-old, and as I hit my late thirties, it's killing me. I can't imagine our two kids and a baby, I'm tired just thinking about it. But my old friend infertility is still with me, and likes to peek out and say hello now and then. I've come to terms that it always will be around, infertility is a part of me—our relationship just changes.

It's been three years since my children's half-brother was born. I'm glad it worked out as it did for all of us and their birth mom. I can't imagine the toll losing Felicia and Chase it has taken on her. I still find myself holding my breath now and then, thinking, *what if something happens?* But I force that out of my mind and try to have faith that she can do this. Like we had predicted, though, he also has challenges, just like our two . . . the genetics are strong. The ability to know about his medical status, though, is a blessing, as he was recently diagnosed with type 1 diabetes. We are going to be getting our children tested to see if they too carry the antibodies that put them at a higher risk of developing diabetes. When you have two children with communication difficulties, it's better know information ahead of time. There are enough unknowns in our life when it comes to the future. Having the ability to know if one or both of my kids are at risk for diabetes gives me peace of mind that we can watch for the signs.

Almost two years into our adoption, we finally received the kid's full CAS files. They are about three inches thick, and contain all the information we were missing. It was like I had finally won the lottery. I had answers to questions I didn't have before, and histories we didn't know about.

We had a general idea about the kids' birth dad from the beginning, but this gave us the grim reality. I came across a family tree of relatives and under the paternal side, and down at the very bottom, it said, "half-sibling—brother." This means, somewhere out there, my children have another half-sibling. There are probably more we don't know about, to be honest. I doubt we will ever know any more information, but he's out there—and I can't help but wonder what that looks like from a disability standpoint. Having the details helps, though—even if it's just a breadcrumb trail.

We have never met our children's birth father, and I don't know if we ever will. Even if we do, we don't plan on allowing our children to have physical access to him. He's made some pretty poor life choices that are extremely unsafe, and I don't want to put my children at risk. My children do know about him, though—and we make sure they know that he is not a bad person. He has just made bad choices, and there were reasons he was the way he was. I would sit in a room with him, though, in a safe space, to ask him questions and try to understand him. Having the ability to understand him would ultimately help me understand my children at a different level. For some reason, I don't worry about CAS calling us randomly to take in a baby from his side.

Maybe I should more? I guess I just always figured we would never know, and part of me is OK with that.

The "baby door" is complicated when you are dealing with infertility, adoption, and special-needs parenting. It's not as simple as choosing not to have another child or having menopause start. I know other special-needs parents who didn't have a choice but to stop after having one child. Having a child with a known genetic disorder often to leads to a higher percentage that a second or third child could also be born with the same condition. Parents who carry these genes need to make the hard decision if they want to risk having more children or not.

Women who go through the process of fertility treatments and then decide not to go any further—that's a hard choice, not taken lightly. When you spent years trying to have a family and don't succeed, but then have the strength to say, "Adoption isn't for me, we aren't going to pursue that life path," I respect it. I don't think I could have made that choice. I am proud to say I have met a few women who did make that choice, and I am a little jealous of the lives that they have created for themselves—but I know that sometimes, it goes both ways.

No one can dictate how you end your journey, and no one can tell you how to feel when you close that "baby door" for the last time.

SIXTEEN:
Mayday, Mayday

"Mommy, it's too loud . . . there are too many people . . . ." Her eyes filled with tears.

Every outing is preplanned. And I don't mean pick a date, pack some snacks, and go. I mean it starts multiple days, weeks, or months in advance. We are hoping to try an amusement park this year—and by that, I mean it's April, and we are already planning for June. We are looking specifically at June, since schools will still be in. We will aim for mid-week, when it's less likely to be overcrowded. Ashley will take the day off, and it'll be a two-on-two ratio. We have read up on the park's accessibility and fast-pass options—so we can avoid any long line wait times if possible and don't even get me started on our children's food intolerance list and trying to accommodate those. We even know how to avoid seeing the waterpark, so the kids don't know it's an option. If we can take out any surprises or anything that we know will cause a meltdown ahead of time, we try our best.

Before trips, we preplan bedtime, to make sure they get enough rest, and we hide any evidence of the trip, since Felicia's anxiety can't handle it. She often doesn't find out until we are already in the truck for long trips. I start packing a week in advance, and hide the suitcases in closets, and our food is pre-ordered for pick up or hiding in bins somewhere in the house. The truck is packed once the kids are in bed or when they are busy. We have it down to an art. We made the mistake of telling her in advance a couple of times, and Felicia sat by the front door and cried for three hours before we left. Not worth it. When we plan a week vacation somewhere we've never been, we've even had to do a short weekend trip there before our actual vacation. Last time we tried to just wing it, Felicia was so anxious and overstimulated that the week was out of control with melt downs and behaviours. We have a system. It doesn't always make sense, but it works.

Summer 2019 had been harder than previous summers . . . . I was more wary about day trips by myself, or who I took with me. I needed people who were calm, cool, and collected and wouldn't get the kids too wound up. The kids were bigger, the meltdowns were bigger, and I couldn't throw them both in a double stroller anymore and exit, stage left. Chase had to be contained due to unsafe running and mobility issues. We had upgraded to a larger jogging stroller for him, which keeps him safe.

It was a beautiful summer day. The kids woke up in great moods. I had been debating visiting a smaller zoo that wasn't too far from home. It was mid-week, which meant less people, and the weather seemed perfect, so I thought, *what the heck, let's do it.* I was feeling confident and ready for a fun day out of the house. Felicia had found out about where we were headed about twenty minutes before we got there and her response was, "But I like the big zoo better." *Tough shit, kid, here we are—and this is what we are doing today.* Kids have such a way of taking all the time and effort trying to bring joy and just squishing it I with a simple sentence, don't they?

We pulled around the corner. The parking lot wasn't full! *Perfect! This should be easy*, I said to myself as I took off my seatbelt. But as I looked up again, I saw them . . . orange shirts *everywhere*. I guess I didn't see the two huge school buses, which only meant one thing . . . summer day camp kids. I slouched back into my seat. *Oh, you've got to be kidding me.* I hadn't thought about the possibility of summer camps in my grand plan.

OK, it'll be fine. Once we get through the gate and inside, we will be fine. I've got this. I unloaded the kids and put Chase in his stroller, and we made our way to the front gate to pay before we headed into the park. Felicia was asking what animals we were going to see, chatting away happily. The moment we crossed the barrier and into the zoo, we were hit with a wall of screaming and the sound of the metal gates to the petting zoo area opening and banging closed. Kids were running everywhere, and the camp staff were yelling—pure chaos, right at the entrance. I was prepared for busy, but I was not prepared for this. I looked down at the tiny face in front of me.

"Mommy, it's too loud, there are too many people . . . ." Her eyes filled with tears, and her hands over her ears. *Mayday, mayday*—we were going down and we hadn't even started yet. We needed to get away from this chaos. I scanned as fast as I could to find somewhere away from the noise and spotted picnic tables in a far corner in the shade. I grabbed her hand as we sped past the animals. We got to the picnic table, and I parked the stroller. Chase was confused about what had just happened, but stayed relaxed. Felicia was instantly done. Her eyes were black from sensory overload. I got down to her level and got her to focus on me counting slowly . . . *one, two, three* . . . before taking a big breath in and letting it out slowly, over and over again. It took ten minutes of calm-down because of one minute of chaos. I sat her on the bench of the picnic table as I rummaged through our bag. Why didn't I have her noise-cancelling headphones? Rookie mistake.

We had two choices: try again to continue with our zoo day, or bail and drive the hour home—which could potentially trigger a bigger, more explosive meltdown, because now, she wanted to be at the zoo. I asked her what she wanted to do, and she decided she wanted to try. I scanned the map and found the most boring animals, where the camp kids would not want to be. Deer—*what rambunctious kid really wants to see deer?*

We did a quick animal tour, looking at the tigers lounging in the sun and the monkeys swinging around, then found a small spot near the deer to try to take a food break. Sometimes, breaks and snacks help. But this time, it was too late. Her anxiety was high, and this this kid refused eat. She never eats well when she's stressed. It was hot, and she was on sensory overload.

"Are there any animals that you want to see?" I asked her. I have to let her feel like she's got some kind of control when she feels that out of control.

"I want to pet the goats," she answered. *Fine*, goats it was. We just needed to end this on a good note, and get out of there in one piece. Sometimes, the goal is just to survive.

As we stood up and got ready to move, Chase began using his sign language, telling me he needed to go pee (the joys of potty-training). *Wait . . . the bathroom . . .* it was over by the screaming camp kids. Now, all I could think was, *please let them have a family bathroom, so we can all fit and stay contained*. We reached the bathroom. I let out a huge sigh of relief as I spotted the accessible bathroom. We all piled into the bathroom, stroller and all. It was cool and quiet, and I looked at both of them.

"Are we ready?" They both said yes.

With a deep breath, we headed in the direction of the goats. I swear to God, the orange shirts had multiplied, and they were everywhere, screaming. The sound of the metal gates opening and slamming closed filled my ears. Felicia was now determined that she was petting a goat . . . *OK, here we go . . . .* Chase wanted out of his stroller and to go into the petting area, too. OK, two loose kids in public—at least they were fenced in. I stood by the gate to make sure neither snuck past me without me seeing. I watched the kids stumble around the small field. Chase tripped over a stick, catching himself before face-planting. Felicia had a goat climbing up her, trying to lick her face, but she was happy. We were doing it. We were successfully petting goats, and I could breathe for a moment.

Normally, transitions are hard. But when I said it was time to go, both kids were more than ready. We negotiated getting out around all the orange shirts, and walked back to the truck. I got into the truck and looked back. Both kids were absolutely spent. Their little faces were drained. Forty-five minutes from the time we got in to the time we got out. Not quite the full afternoon I had planned, but no one had gotten violent or laid on the ground. We made it. I feel like I had gotten lucky, and it was an incredibly quiet drive home.

As we flew by in the far end of the zoo before we left, I did notice you, though, mama. Through our chaos, I saw you standing by the monkeys. I always notice the moms like me. I saw the strain in your eyes as your little boy was "hand-flapping" and jumping with excitement. I saw you, also, watching the orange shirts, on high alert, and I smiled in solidarity, knowing you and your little boy were doing your absolute best to be in the community, just like us. But I also smiled because you had remembered the headphones....

If we don't take chances, we will never see anything in the world. My kids can't just turn off autism. Sensory overload is real. They struggle, and I struggle to help them—no matter how prepared we are. What we gauge as a successful outing doesn't always match a neurotypical family. The zoo was an "iffy" day, but we made it. Sometimes, it feels like teetering on a high wire, trying not to let anyone fall, while weighing your choices of what's just enough and what will send them over the edge.

During our home study during the start of the adoption process, we had wrote down on our paper that we weren't ready for parenting a child with autism, and at the ARE, we avoided profiles with autism listed. I knew plenty of families who had a child with autism, and even have various family members with different disabilities, including my cousin, who also has autism. She has grown up to be an amazing woman, who is smart, creative, and hilarious. That's totally our phenomenal genetics. Ashley wasn't as exposed to people with disabilities throughout her life as I had been. She didn't feel like she had the knowledge, understanding, patience or confidence to adopt a child with a disability—especially the needs autism can require. It can sometimes be an overwhelming two-foot jump into the world of special needs. It turns out the universe was laughing at us, and had another plan.

When Chase was diagnosed with autism and his global developmental delay was upgraded to an intellectual disability, I knew it was coming—and it still hit me harder than I was expecting.

Felicia was diagnosed as soon as we could get it done. I knew way before we had the official report in our hands. I had fought for the diagnosis. With Chase, it had been different. This little man had been through it all already in his little life. He was born at twenty-eight weeks at three pounds with a grade-one hole in his heart, and blind until he was eight months old. He didn't sit on his own until he was sixteen months, start to crawl until nineteen months, and wasn't walking until well into his second year. He was then diagnosed with cerebellar hypoplasia, and he has a genetic abnormality—but in his own time, he's progressed, slowly. When he was four years old, we noticed the developmental gap widen, as he still wasn't talking. We were suspecting the possibility of apraxia—or it was the cerebellar hypoplasia. We had his hearing test, to rule out a hearing impairment. I am an all-cards-on-the-table kind of person—give me all the information so I can make a plan—especially with two complex children. When we brought him home, the future was filled with possibilities of verbal communication and catching up to his peers. When he was diagnosed with autism, I suddenly had reality hit me. This child had so many things stacked against him—like a wall he had to climb over—how were we going to tackle it all with both children?

In our house, there is no such thing as a break from autism especially with two children. We have days that we are barely surviving, other days one child will be happy, and the other isn't, and on the rare day both children are having a good day and we are ready to tackle the world. There are days we can safely leave the house, and others, the battle just seems too great. As the children have grown, Felicia especially has been able to label where she is struggling and ask for help. She has all the tools for coping, and most of the time, she uses them—which is a huge improvement, and it's everything you want your child to be able to do. Some things are getting easier, and some harder, as she strives for independence—as all children try to do. I used to look at parents with multiple kids with autism and think, *Man, that's hard. I'm so glad that's not us* . . . . Joke's on me—we've been those people all along.

There are days I watch Felicia play in the backyard—and by play, I mean throwing pinecones into the blow-up pool as she laughs. There is absolutely no functional play—she's just stimming. Some days, I try to encourage more structure than others—but as long as she's not being destructive, we let it happen . . . you pick your battles. When we go to the store, she runs for the baby toys. They are bright, loud, and tend to play music—a sensory child's dream. I used to try to deter her, toward more age-appropriate toys—but that was my own insecurity. Now, I just let her. What's it hurting, anyway? I think that's a part of accepting where your child is in life. Felicia has no idea how to entertain herself. She needs to be guided and told what to do all the time—and if she's not doing a structured activity, it's just pure chaos, or she walks around, lost.

Ashley Biddiscombe

Chase is more engaged with pretend play—he will keep himself busy for hours, as long as he's in arm's reach of me. But when things don't go perfectly as planned, or a Hot Wheels car is out of place in his very organized line, you can guarantee something is getting thrown. He has a whole pretend world, and I wish I knew what he was saying, so I could be let in a little more. He loves cars, stuffed animals, and the play kitchen. They are skills we never thought he would have, and they change every day.

They have been trying to play hide-and-seek together lately, though. They need help, but they are doing it in their own way—and that's pretty special.

Recently, things started to change with Chase. He's been less focused on tasks and moving much faster, which I didn't think was possible. His meltdowns are bigger and more explosive. His behaviour is erratic and impulsive. He's flushed things down the toilet. He piles things into a big, heaping pile in his room that makes no sense to us—but it does to him. He's broken things in the house without a blink of an eye or remorse, and he barely sleeps. He is up at the crack of dawn, moving constantly from the time his feet hit the floor to late into the night. Even in his bed, exhausted, he cannot seem to calm his body. I started suspecting ADHD, but I was also getting triggered back to the early days with Felicia and prayed we weren't regressing. We went back to the psychologist for an update on his psychological assessment, and my gut was right . . . ADHD. Even though I went looking for the diagnosis so we could get help, staring at that official piece of paper cut through me.

When you are living the day to day, you forget how complex the kids are on paper. They have come so far in daily life, but the intricacies in each of their five diagnoses are sometimes mind-blowing. Sometimes, I just need to sit in the grief for a day, feel it, accept it—and then I can move on. And this was one of those times.

Ashley and I took the report to the doctor. It was time to ask for help. We don't seek medication for many things, and heading down this new road was not an easy decision. There is no way this struggling little boy feels good in this state, and I can feel myself slowly burning out trying to keep up with him and stay ahead of the destruction, always feeling two steps behind. We will do anything we can to help our kids. It's new territory for us, but we will figure it out, and get help for our son and our family.

SEVENTEEN:
Labels

Several years ago, I had a conversation with a couple whose child had been "having a challenging time" for a while. In our gut, Ashley and I knew what it was—but you can't tell other parents what you suspect their child has unless they are ready to hear it. We talked about testing, diagnosing, and specialists, and the husband's response was "I don't want to put a label on my child." He wasn't ready for the commitment that it entailed, and accepting what that meant.

During our adoption process, our children were great unknowns—no formal diagnosis, and no real answers. Our kid's foster mom was phenomenal—she knew what the kids needed—but her hands were also tied to the system. When a child is in foster care, their official guardian is the CAS, and no diagnostics can be ordered unless the CAS put the request in. There are too many in care and not enough workers, so kids fall through the cracks. Once we had guardianship, nothing was going to stop me from getting answers. I'd find every specialist if it meant resources and help. For me, there is a power in knowledge. So I will fill my brain with everything I need to know, so I can attack a problem from all angles.

Getting a child diagnosed takes work, and it can be scary with so many unfamiliar faces and specialists. Parents aren't always ready to jump into the unknown. The unknown means change, and change can be overwhelming. The family as whole needs to be on board and ready to accept the information. Though people are afraid of labels for their children, they get you help. They get you resources and your children help at school, sometimes extra funding to go towards therapy or respite care. Labels aren't always a bad thing. A child who has hearing aids, a wheelchair, or a walker has a physical sign of their disability. Their labels are out in the world from the moment they are given these tools. However, their parents need to fight the stigmas that surround them, convincing society that their child can thrive despite their disability. Children who have "invisible disabilities" are those with intellectual disabilities, social disorders, ADHD, trauma, and other disabilities you cannot physically see. Those children need those labels so that they can be given the resources to thrive in the world. These diagnostic labels have gotten us early intervention, occupational therapists, speech therapists, physiotherapy, social workers, psychologists, neurologists, geneticists, specialized social programs, respite, funding options . . . . We couldn't be where we are today without all those tools, and I'm grateful for all the people who have helped us along the way.

In our house, we use the term "special needs" when generalizing our children's diagnoses. Some families don't like that term, and disabled adults tend to prefer to identify as "disabled" and not "special needs." Many parents use the term "special needs" when referring to their child with a disability—especially when their child is in the early stages of their diagnosis. They aren't ready to say, "my child is disabled," which tends to go hand in hand with the parent's level of acceptance of the information that they are trying to process.

Ashley Biddiscombe

If I was to turn to someone and say, "Oh, my daughter with autism, intellectual disability, ADHD, attachment disorder, and my son with cerebellar hypoplasia, autism intellectual disability, ADHD, and speech delay. Oh, and both children have and genetic abnormality on gene ZMIZ1," people would look at me like I was nuts. So, we choose to blanket the diagnoses and just say we have two children with special needs. If someone asks for more information, we are happy to share.

There are families that prefer to say that they have "a child with autism," and some prefer "an autistic child." The important thing is that when that child grows up and knows more about their own diagnosis, they get to choose how they want to be identified. For example, Felicia may grow up and say, "Hi, I am Felicia, and I have autism." She may prefer to say, "Hi, I am Felicia, and I am autistic." Whatever way she wants to claim identity within her diagnosis is completely up to her.

Our children are more than their diagnoses, and we advocate every day for quality education, inclusion, and acceptance. Our children have the ability to learn new things, participate in recreation, thrive in community groups, make friends, love and be loved. Their progression may not look the same as another child their age, but even the smallest thing they achieve can be cause for the biggest celebration. As humans, we are lifelong learners—and children like to prove the world wrong with the things that they can do.

Chase is seven years old, and with his diagnosis, he really shouldn't be able to run, climb, and jump, but he shows us every day that characteristics of cerebellar hypoplasia will not define him. He is now just starting to express himself verbally, and if someone says,

"Will he ever fully talk?" I smile and I say,

"I don't know," because I honestly don't. He surprises us every day with the things he can do—and I'm here to help him achieve whatever he can.

Felicia's level of intellectual disability creates learning difficulties—especially in sequencing—but if she meets someone for the first time, she will remember their name forever. And don't ever question her ability to remember a name—she will prove you wrong every time. Her memory is impeccable with names and faces.

There are not too many children who can name almost all the countries in Asia by their shape . . . she can. She excels at shapes, in fact. One day, I was watching her do a puzzle upside down, which confused me. Most people look at the image right side up, and the details of each puzzle piece that they are searching for.

She looked up at me and said, "Mommy, I need one that looks like half a heart."

"OK, what colours are on the piece?" I started shuffling around the box, and she looked at me like she had no idea what I was talking about.

"No, it just needs to look like it half a heart." She pointed down. Her brain only saw the shapes she needed, no other details. She did a one-hundred-and-fifty-piece puzzle by just looking at shapes. I don't think I could've done that. Just because someone doesn't see the world the same way that you do doesn't mean that they are wrong.

As a parent of two children who see the world in their own distinct way, I am taught new, abstract ways of seeing the world that I never would have dreamed of. I also don't have a choice sometimes. If I can't see what they are seeing or can't understand what they are trying to explain to me, I hear about it—and not quietly, I might add. In order adapt to your children's world, you have to flex yourself and your thinking in ways that you never imagined possible—and I am thankful for those perspectives, because they honestly make me a better person.

When I was teaching riding, I would watch children and adults of all ages get onto horses. Most children would sit up in the saddle, with volunteers on one or both sides of them, fearless, like they could take on the world. Some children we would lay down on a soft pad if their bodies didn't allow them to sit. There were children with trach tubes, body bracing, leg bracing. Some used hearing aids, guide dogs, canes, walkers, and wheelchairs. Not one child coming through those doors let their disability keep them from getting on a horse. We would work on balance, sitting quietly, steering, independent. Sometimes, a small skill, like leaning forward and touching the horse's neck, was a *huge* skill— due to balance or muscle tightness. When they finally did it, we all cheered, because we knew how hard they had worked to achieve it. Their parents brought them, week to week, allowing them the opportunity to be a part of a group and feel pride—and no one cared what label their disability had. We just wanted everyone to succeed, whatever that meant for them. I miss teaching. I miss being around the most amazing people I have ever met in my life. But with the stage we are at now and the busyness of our life at home, I can't do everything. Maybe one day, I will be back in the arena. But for now, I just need to watch from the sidelines.

When Felicia started swimming with the Special Olympic recreation program, she was the smallest child in the pool. There were kids older than her, and many adults—mainly with down syndrome—who were participating. Every week, we would head out on a Friday night for our big night of swimming. As a society, we tend to veer away from people who are different than us. We learn that *different* can be scary and unknown. Felicia, like any child, has questions about other people—but she has this ability to accept everyone just as they are, and move on. Among her peers, she sees no difference, and will talk and interact with anyone she's allowed to—even if they can't talk back. She will throw a ball to another person in the pool and befriend anyone that will let her. At swimming, she loves to race against a lady much older than herself. She doesn't see someone with down syndrome—she sees someone to race with, laugh with, and swim with. When you stop and truly watch children with disabilities you soon realize as a society we could learn a lot from their strength, determination, love, and acceptance of others. They tend to live without too many fears, and live life more fully than we may ever do as adults.

When our children end up with their first or even their fifth diagnosis, it doesn't change who they are. I've heard the sentence "I don't know how you do it—I don't think I could—you've got a lot on your plate" so many times over the years by different people in our lives.

However, the baby that you held and rocked to sleep every night, the toddler that you pushed in the swings at the park, the child that just lost their first tooth . . . you aren't just suddenly parenting a child with a diagnosis. You've been parenting them all along. That diagnosis—that label—is going to help get you the tools for your child you didn't have access to before. But that child hasn't changed one bit. I think that it is hard to pull back and look at the whole, grand scheme of things—especially when emotions are running high, you are grieving, and you are in "the hard."

I heard someone say once that everyone has a lot on their plate, but not everyone has the same plate. Meaning, maybe my full plate is a strong, ceramic platter that can hold a lot of things, but maybe my friend's plate is a flimsy paper plate that can only take on small things—otherwise, theirs will fall apart, and they would drop everything to the ground. Sometimes, we choose our plates depending on what we have going on in our lives—and sometimes, we wish we could put our plates down. It's not that you are weak or less than someone else, it just means that's what you can handle at the time—and it's OK to say, "I can't do this right now."

Ashley Biddiscombe

Ash and I go back and forth with our patience, tolerance, and abilities all the time. Sometimes, she can load more on her plate and pick up the slack when I am struggling, and sometimes I put more on my plate and pick up the slack. The hard part for both of us is admitting when we are struggling. We are both too stubborn. On the days we both have paper plates—well, those are the days that the house is in chaos, we are sitting on the couch binge-watching a show series, and we order in food. We have our limits, just like everyone else.

EIGHTEEN:
Alone in a Crowded Room

Have you ever felt completely alone in a crowded room?

Being the only gay couple in amongst most of our friends and family for a long time wasn't always easy. Our relationship journey was different than our other friend couples. We can sit among other married couples and share similar experiences, but there is still the fact we are two women sitting around heterosexual couples. Other couples didn't have to "come out," they didn't have to worry about acceptance or if someone would be willing to marry them. They don't have to worry about where they go on vacation and their safety. They get to live life in a society that is predominantly straight. We've often sat in rooms where people have made homophobic remarks or jokes with zero sensitivity that we are sitting there, not cluing into the fact they are making fun of the people in community that we are apart of. As a queer couple, we must make the choice to stand up and say, "Hey, not cool," or sit there and let it slide depending on who we are dealing with—and that choice isn't always easy. Society tends to see two women together as "more acceptable" than two men or someone who is transgender, due to the over sexualization of women. Ashley and I conditioned ourselves early in our relationship not to hold hands or kiss each other in front of other people for their comfort level, not ours, and in some cases depending on where we are, for our safety. Even though society is changing, we still have a long way to go, and homophobia is everywhere.

When we were going through fertility treatments, I would sit in the waiting room, waiting to be called back to be poked and prodded, and I would look around the room. If I caught eyes with another woman, we would both quickly look away. We were on our own journeys, but going through the exact same thing—but no one talked or acknowledged each other. When I created my first blog post and sent it out into the world, I had three ladies message me within a day—they had thought they, too, were alone in infertility. No one talked about the struggle, no one talked about the pain, we all just kept our tears behind closed doors and moved through life. It would have been so much easier if we had all just gone through the ups and downs together, saying the things to each other that we couldn't say to anyone else.

Sitting at PRIDE training at a table with two other couples, learning, talking, laughing, and sometimes holding back tears, gave us a sense of community we hadn't had until that moment. But we were still *the gay couple*, and some of the things we had to think about with adoption were different. Every time we filled out paperwork for the children, or someone new came into our lives, it was like coming out all over again.

Once we adopted, I realized the amazing support that was available to adoptive parents—support groups in person, online, resources, social workers running therapy groups. But in the special-needs world, the parent support isn't as widespread as I had thought it was—and finding a group that supports parents with special needs children and that were adopted . . . now, you are really digging deep.

Special needs parents sit in waiting rooms together, smiling, saying hi. We ask casually about each other's kids, but rarely does it go deeper than that. We are all in the same space—but on our own islands with our own struggles—we do not compare notes and check in.

Many adaptive classes—depending on the sport—run at the same time as regular classes. You find yourself in changerooms, or a viewing lounge, and you have the only special needs child in the bunch. As the parents around you talk about their child's friends, sleepovers, and accomplishments, you sit there thinking about speech therapy from that morning, and how your child doesn't have any friends—and again, you are alone in a crowded room. We have made this cozy little world for our two kids. I often forget about the outside world that we aren't really a part of.

Felicia, at an early age, took to the world of gymnastics, which has been amazing for her sensory needs, strength, balance, and determination. We get to go to our adaptive program at our local gymnastics centre. She loves her coach, and she is thriving. One session, one of her classes were at the same time as a tot and a mom/dad class. I am normally full blinders on when we are out. I don't always notice who is around us. My focus tends to be on anything that may trigger a meltdown and my children's cues of functioning in the environment.

This day specific day, though, we walked into the building, and I saw the crowd of parents and kids. There was a baby crying, the kids were in the hallway talking away to their parents as they removed their shoes and coats—basically, a typical tot class. I stood and assessed the situation carefully. Toddlers were everywhere, noise was echoing in the halls. My brain automatically goes to *how do I get her through without sending her into sensory overload before we even get into the gym?*

I started taking her outdoor gear off in the lobby instead of the coat rack. I put her noise-cancelling headphones on, and then I got down to her level and looked her in the eyes. I could see her already starting to drain from the commotion as I talked her through the next steps of getting through the crowd.

"Hold mommy's hand. We are going to go past everyone and find your teacher. You are OK. The noise will be better when you get in." These quick preplanning sessions come natural now—I don't even think about it. My eyes raised, and I looked up and see a mom of one of the young girls staring at us. I'm sure it was just a curious stare, as they normally are, but for some reason on this day, it made me feel out of place. I ushered Felicia through the crowd as quick as I could, but then I became hyper-aware of the fact every parent I passed was now watching my now-stimming child as she got excited to go in with her coach.

I tried to get my head back into the game as I handed over Felicia to her coach. I sat down to watch Felicia, but my eyes wandered over at the tot class—these little, tiny humans climbing, rolling, and balancing so easily, without having to think about their movements—and I found myself holding back tears. My kids had come so far—but it's those moments I realized how different we were as a family. At the time, Chase was four years old, and nowhere near the physical ability of these two-year-olds. The skills that they were producing in front of my eyes far surpassed Chase's. Every milestone, big or small, in our house, is celebrated, because it takes *soooo* long for the kids to learn new skills. Hell, I was ready to break out the wine when Chase started saying "do do do." It took forever to get the *d* sound. It's funny how your interpretation of success changes.

I watched my little girl in the corner away from any other parents. I didn't feel like having the "how old is your daughter" conversation. She was jumping, swinging, and balancing, happy as could be, and I reminded myself that she was participating right alongside the other children, and that was to be celebrated.

Around this same time, Chase was in his no-sleep pattern—something we had been experiencing since he had come home. He would go weeks where he would not sleep through the night, nor nap. He would wake up crying multiple times, much like an infant—and he would often go through the days with less than four hours of solid sleep. The less sleep he got, the less coordinated his already-uncoordinated body became. The moment anything didn't work for him, you could see the rage start all the way down in his toes and rise like a thermometer though his body. His whole body would shake and turn bright red, and we would wait for the "The Hulk" to come out, in the biggest, longest scream he could muster, followed by him normally throwing whatever was available. He gained the nickname "Baby Hulk." I would often tell the therapists about these episodes, but they never saw them. They only saw happy-go lucky Chase, or a of glimmer of his temper, which always quickly dissipated when distracted.

One day, we were at the centre for physiotherapy, and we had his physiotherapist, occupational therapist, and the social worker all in the room. They had all been with us since the beginning, and were our therapy family—which tends to happen when therapists are the only adults you see in a week. They wanted to try Chase out on a treadmill, to stabilize his walking. We were about two weeks into a non-sleep cycle, and I gave them the heads-up the moment we arrived.

"He hasn't slept in two weeks. He's been raging the last couple of days."

"Naps?" his occupational therapist asked.

"None. He just lays there, vocally stimming, nonstop, '*eeee ya eee ya eee ya.*'" She nodded as she looked at his tiny blonde head and tired eyes, trying to make a plan to keep him motivated.

The physiotherapist hooked him into a harness that would keep his body in the centre of the treadmill so if he fell it would catch him, and keep him from injuring himself. Our occupational therapist was there to encourage him and give him breaks in between the spans of demanding work. He had the strongest connection to her and would do basically anything she asked. The social worker was with me, watching from the sidelines. She was doing the "how are you doing?" check-in with me, which I always greatly appreciated. She was one of the few people I could be honest with, and she never tried to fix things. She just listened.

The therapists turned on the treadmill at the slowest pace and tried to encourage him to walk. Chase took a few steps. then tried to fall to his knees in protest, the harness catching him. *Come on, buddy, you can do this.* They stopped, readjusted, then started again. He flung his head back in protest again, letting his feet get pushed back by the treadmill before lifting them up, refusing to participate. He was only about thirty pounds, which wasn't a lot of weight in the harness, and he let his body swing around, with his head back, not caring about what they wanted him to do. Now that he knew he could just lift his legs and not participate in the activity, it was no longer going to happen. They took him out and took a break.

Chase is the king of shortcuts. If he can find a way to make any task easier and not do it to the fullest, he will, every time. This wasn't the first time they were being outsmarted by him. During the physiotherapy block before this one, they had tried to get him to walk up and down a padded ramp to work on his balance. They would put a toy up at the top, then get him to walk up, grab the toy, and bring it back down the ramp. After the second time getting to the top, he promptly sat down on the platform and threw all the toys down the ramp. He then got up, walked one last time down the ramp, and handed them to the therapists. I sat, dying of laughter. He was delayed, but not stupid. The therapists looked at me, shaking their heads.

They put him back on the treadmill without the harness and stayed close to support him. He took a few steps and then basically let them catch him before he fell. This wasn't going to happen today—there was no point in pushing it. They sat him down on the floor with a large peg board—one we had used a million times before. You can stack brightly-coloured pegs and make tall towers. Chase loved this activity, and it was a good break to regroup.

He sat there pushing the pegs together as we chatted about a plan to get him moving. Suddenly, his mood changed as I watched. His hands that were clearly not cooperating with what he wanted them to do, and I watched his face start to turn red. *Oh shit, here comes Baby Hulk.* The occupational therapist tried to help him, showing him it was OK, and they could work together, but he wasn't having it. His body began to shake in anger, he screamed in a way he had never screamed before, and he stood up, dumping all hundred pegs on the floor, then turned to a small therapy table and flipped it over. His rage was spilling from every ounce of his body. The room stopped and stared, not sure what to do with this version of him. Before he could continue with his damage rampage, I grabbed him quickly and laid him on the floor. I crawled over top of him, on all fours, my body acting as a barrier and stabilizer against his little, raging body. He laid between my hands and legs, my face inches above his.

"Chase, Chase . . . look at Mommy. Breathe . . . come on, buddy, let's count . . ." I slowly and rhythmically counted, "One, two, three, four . . ." until I hit thirty. "Deep breath." There was something about the vocal sound of counting that always seemed to work with the children, like a metronome musicians use to keep time—constant, steady, and calm. His eyes met mine. My little boy was back, but he was spent. That was a lot of energy he just sent into the universe.

I raised my eyes, not sure how long we had been counting for. All the therapists were sitting on therapy bed now, watching us, not sure how they should help. In that moment, in a room of people that knew my little boy the best, with all their collective knowledge, they didn't know how to help him or me. No one had answers to help his sleep problems, which led to his rage, which led to damage and self-harm. It was us, figuring it out all on our own.

I've realized how special the adaptive world can be. I realized just how special it is to be around other people who "get it" without having to say a word. Even though we are all on our own islands of "hard," sitting silently in a crowded room, we are still in our little cocoon of safety. Where noise-cancelling headphones aren't weird, meltdowns happen, and stimming means joy. Parents sit in the waiting rooms of therapy centres and recreation programs, and we are still doing it together, supporting each other—and that glance across the room can mean more than any word ever spoken.

I've also realized the importance of getting our children out into the community. For decades, children with disabilities were locked away in institutions—and now, we have an opportunity to create inclusion. Tolerance and acceptance of those different than us starts with exposure at an early age. When we create programs that are inclusive or run side-by-side neurotypical children and able-bodied children, we create a more inclusive environment—therefore, children can learn from each other instead of avoiding one another. By educating our children on how we are the same and how our differences are not scary, we are also creating advocates. These younger generations are going to be adults alongside our children with disabilities, and the work we put in while they are all young will ultimately create a better world when they all grow up. So, instead of feeling like I need to hide and protect my children from the stares we get in public, I look at it as: *we are spreading disability awareness everywhere we go.*

My son has leg braces to help him walk, and he has a speech device that gives him a clear voice to communicate. My daughter sometimes has noise-cancelling headphones, and sometimes needs to be reminded about her social skills. Take the time to talk to your children about the tools children with disabilities need to help them succeed—and if you aren't sure, ask. Most parents willingly tell you what their children's tools are for—just like your child might need training wheels on their bike or a comfort stuffed animal in strange places, my child uses a speech device to help him talk. As adults, we don't give children enough credit for what they can process—their questions are often purely out of curiosity, because someone looks different than them, or different from what they see at home.

As a parent, when you can make that shift from feeling alone in a crowded room to the acceptance that your family may look different, it changes how you feel about everything.

At the end of the day, we are all doing mass amounts of laundry, staring at the sink full of dirty dishes, and kissing our children goodnight. We really aren't all that different from one another. We are all just doing the best we can to make sure we keep our children alive and to make sure that they don't turn into assholes when they grow up.

NINETEEN: Marriage

Let's put this out there: I am no marriage expert, and I will never claim to be. We are celebrating twelve years of marriage, together for eighteen—which is like toddler years in the grand scheme of life. It is, however, amazing what can happen in over a decade. I feel like I have packed in enough adulting already for a lifetime.

There are so many things I wish we had known before this journey. The number of crossroads we have stopped at, choosing to go left, right, or turn back around. The decisions we've had to make together and separately. The fights, the tears, the happiness, the small moments, and the big.

I think back to our wedding. It was exactly what we wanted it to be. It was fun, light—something for people to enjoy and celebrate with us. We were young, and had no idea of the path that would be laid out in front of us. Life before infertility, before heartbreak, death, grieving, adoption, depression, and disabilities. We didn't know how a marriage could be tested so many times and in so many ways. There have been times I wasn't sure if we'd make it—and we maybe almost didn't.

Love isn't like the movies, or like people portray on social media. No one tells you that sometimes, you just feel like roommates, and you must choose every day to love someone. No one tells you that can fall out of love, and you sometimes must fight to fall back in love. You don't realize how experiences change you, and you can either choose to grow together or drift apart—and how hard it can be to hold on.

I read a post today about how the qualities you look for in a spouse when you are young change as you get older, and it's amazing how true that is. When you're young, you search for someone, you are attracted to and have the same interests, maybe seems stable in life . . . is there much more to go off of when you're young? After being in the trenches of marriage, it is so much incredibly deeper than that. It's all the small things that truly make the bigger picture. Of course, we all want happiness and good times, but you need someone who you know is there for "the hard." Find someone who is there for the bad, no matter what. The person who sits with you on the kitchen floor while you bawl your eyes out—and I mean the ugly-cry-with-snot-dripping-down-your-face kind of cry—and says you'll get through it together.

The person you can message during the day and say, "this has been one hell of a day," and they come home with a bottle of wine and M&Ms without you asking.

The person who lets you sleep in and gets up with the kids on a Saturday morning.

The person who isn't afraid of explosive diapers, fevers, and kid vomit, and is up in the middle of the night with you helping to clean it off the top bunk of a bunkbed (trust me, the bunkbed is the highest test at three in the morning).

The person who admits some of their favourite clothing choices are ones you'd never be caught dead in public in, and tells you they love you when you haven't showered and are in the dry-shampoo stage.

The person you can sit and binge watch TV with without any expectations of getting anything done. Did I rope her into fifteen seasons of *ER*? Yes, yes, I did—and she didn't laugh at me while I cried a full three episodes before Dr. Greene died.

The person who sends you out for a day by yourself and has no problem picking up the slack with the kids and the house.

The person who has compassion for people, for animals, and for the elderly.

The person who respects your passions and dreams, even if they aren't theirs—or understands yours.

The person who picks apart every detail of an autism meltdown to figure out how you can deal with it better, and never misses the big meetings for your kids.

The person who randomly takes a day off work to go to the zoo with you.

A person who is always striving to be better for you, the kids, and your family.

The person who still leaves you "I love you" post-it notes for you to find in the morning. For the record, this is not me—I fail at romantic gestures.

The person who admits their flaws and still loves you for yours.

The one thing I know is that Ash and I are better as a team at everything we do. The kids, construction projects, chores, dreams. We take pride in having an open door to anyone who needs it, and it's just an unspoken agreement that if someone needs help, we open the door first and ask questions later. We even help people get better together. We love our strays—people and animals . . . we really aren't all that picky. We take pride that our house can act as a safe haven.

Some ideas are crazier than others, but somehow, we get it done or tackle it, even when the other is going, "What the hell were you thinking?". . . . *Ahem*, adopting two kids with special needs sound familiar? I'm just kidding . . . or am I?

We are moving into the next stage, and I am excited for that. The kids are getting bigger, and the house I so desperately wanted to fill at the start is getting smaller. We are putting together plans for a larger house, where we can work and live, that the kids can grow into with us and gain independence in. It's sad to think about leaving this little semi-detached. We started everything in this house—our biggest make-it-or-break-it moments. If we don't take this next step, we may all kill each other. I have a feeling we will plan this whole thing out the same way we did our wedding—clear-cut and efficient, with some bumps along the way—and probably a lot of swearing.

Our marriage will grow and change again, I am sure, but we are going into this as the team we've always been. Marriage starts at the altar, but it's everything you choose in between that will make or break you. Every day, you need to *choose* to love—it doesn't always just happen. Find your teammate, your ride-or-die partner in crime. The two girls who stood at the base of the tree and said their vows so many years ago were just babies. We were hopeful, determined, and had no idea what we were doing. Today, we still don't know what we are doing. We are making it up as we go. It's a hard realization when you go looking for the marriage manual and it doesn't exist.

If I had a choice to do over this life and redesign our path, there are a few things I would change—but I can honestly say I would pick her, every time. We still have work to do to be better for ourselves and each other, but aren't we always a work in progress as humans? The saying "aging like fine wine" exists for a reason—and I really like a good wine. If we had it right all the time, life would be pretty boring. Just because it gets hard sometimes doesn't mean it's over—it's just a chapter in your story. If, for some reason, it is over and you can't make it work, that's OK, too—you haven't failed. We only get one life to live. Live it to its fullest, no matter what that looks like—and if you can create a village of people around you who support you, then you will succeed.

TWENTY:
Healing through Art

Self-care. I think it's one of the most cringe-worthy terms when you are a parent. All the professionals throw the term around like it's easy to do.

"You should really make time for self-care . . . ." Insert eye-roll here. Your brain automatically goes toward long, luxurious baths and pampering at the spa. I can barely remember which day it is or which child needs a bath tonight, and don't ask me if I switched the laundry around because I probably didn't.

As a society, we have been brainwashed to think that our basic human needs equal self-care, such as showering, eating a meal, using the bathroom—as if doing these tasks alone is the ultimate reward. However, sometimes self-care is taking a deeper look inside yourself, facing the good, bad, and the ugly in order to heal. Self-care can be reading a book, doing something you love, and reconnecting with yourself. Everyone's self-care is different, and there is no formula for this. I will say it again, though: your basic needs as a human do not count as luxuries. Self-care is not a luxury—it's a basic need for your own mental health and overall wellbeing. It took me a long time to accept this—but once you realize it, you will never go back.

I used to get up and rush to get ready, thinking the moment the children's eyes opened, they had to be tended to. I would be stressed before the day even began. Now, one of my self-care moments is getting myself ready in my time before I get the kids up and moving. It's not the act of showering or brushing my teeth—it's doing it at my pace and in silence. Taking away the stress of what is happening on the other of the door allows me to get into a good mental space to start the day. We somehow got lucky with our children—they play in their rooms in the morning and don't come out to start the day until we get them. Maybe we trained them this way? Either way, I get up, I shower, I get dressed, and I go through my routine. I take a deep breath, and then start their day. They are safe and happy, playing away in their rooms. When I open their doors, I am normally greeted with their smiling faces, and we all get our breakfast ready. Honestly, it changed everything for my mental health in the morning, and I no longer feel like I'm running to catch up. That one slight change to my routine made life more manageable.

When you have a trauma in your life of any kind, you need to accept that it changes you as a person. Your perspective of the world around you and aspects of yourself change. One of my traumas is what we went through with infertility and the treatments that went along with it. For me, giving this trauma a voice, for other people to know they aren't alone, has given me new life—but it took reaching deep within myself to be able to start to heal. Healing is a process . . . . I still feel the sting with pregnancy announcements, and have a challenging time being around women who are pregnant, no matter how close they are to me—for some reason, it's hard to lock it away. I can hold babies now and it does not feel like my heart is going to ache so hard it will break from my chest . . . small steps, small wins. When we adopted the kids, it threw me into something new. I didn't have to think about what had happened to me physically, mentally, and emotionally. But all unresolved feelings and thoughts have a way of resurfacing when you least expect it.

When I was working, I felt as though I always had a purpose, that my job was greater than I could imagine. When we brought the children home, I lost something that had made me . . . well, *me*. I lost all parts of myself, really. They were all poured into what the children needed. I was even pouring when there was nothing left to pour.

A few years ago, I decided I needed to do something I liked again. I couldn't go back to work with the demands of our life, but there were things I could do at home during naptimes that were just mine. I started painting for fun at first—an easy way to satisfy my creative side that I had been desperately missing. Growing up, I loved art class. When I wasn't in a class, I was drawing and painting at home or doing some sort of craft. Once I was out on my own, I stopped. Adulting took over, and I put the paint brushes away. Taking them back out was intimidating at first, but once I started playing around with figurative art on canvas, it sparked a part of my brain that I had forgotten about. I would paint the figures and see what they would turn into, without pressure or expectation. One day, I was painting a woman—her face was turned away, sitting in a calm position—and it just felt different. I couldn't pinpoint why she mesmerized me so much, and then one day, I looked up at the image and I felt it: the girl was me. I named her "Finding Stillness." She was what I was searching so desperately for. She sold a couple years later. I was sad to see her go, but the woman who bought her fell in love with her, just as I had. It's weird having my inner thoughts and feelings staring me in the face, literally—a representation of the good, the bad, and the ugly finally coming out in a way I wasn't expecting. I found a way to work through things that I was feeling, and the key was my paintbrush.

It takes a lot more strength to pick up a paintbrush and just let it all go than I realized. When I work on a piece now, I am fully aware of what I feel in the moment. I have promised myself that

I will let myself feel what I need to when I paint. Sometimes, I work fast, and feel the joy the piece gives me—and admittedly sometimes, there are tears, and it takes longer to get the figure on the canvas. Sometimes, I have to put a piece away half-done, and come back to it when I'm in a specific mood—but it's part of the process. The harder pieces I hold onto a little tighter, letting the finished image stay on my easel for a few days until I'm ready to let her go into the world. The deeper I go into my own self, the more I let go—and the more I realize what I want and don't want in my life to make me happier. I never thought that I could heal through art, and creating the "Woman Series" has pushed me further artistically, mentally, and emotionally than I could have ever imagined. It is my form of self-care. For me, art has a way of healing the soul. I just had to be open to the possibility.

There are some weeks I don't get down into my studio and pieces get left for a while. I can see other people constantly creating on social media, and I am jealous of their stamina, but then I remind myself it's not a competition. Once I can muster up the energy and time, I close the door behind me, blast some early 2000s alternative rock, and get lost in my own little world. I have to make a conscious effort to put myself in the studio—sometimes, walking through the door is the hardest part. Creativity always follows, and I always come out a better person than the one who walked in.

My message to you is to find that thing that brings you joy and let yourself fall into them. Stop making excuses. The dishes and laundry can wait—we all know they won't go anywhere. Self-care is like putting your oxygen mask on first. How can you teach your child to be whole person if you aren't one yourself? You are in charge of your own happiness. You are in control of your mental and emotional wellbeing. You cannot continually give up everything for everyone else and leave nothing for yourself. You will crash, you will burn out—and then who are you good for?

TWENTY-ONE:
The Not-So-Accessible World

A few weeks ago, I brought Felicia to the mall for the first time in years—and that's not an exaggeration. With our world at a standstill with the pandemic, and the various stages she had been at with her sensory needs, it had literally been years. We had finished up at speech therapy and had some time to kill before another appointment, so with the mall around the corner, I thought, *Why don't we try to get some lunch?* Felicia loves being out, and the thought of going to the mall was just as exciting as if I had said "Let's go to Disney."

"OK, if it's too loud, though, we will get our food and bring it back to the truck." We were sitting in the truck in the parking lot, making our clear plan before going in.

"But it won't be too loud—we can eat in the mall." She was adamant this was going to happen.

"I know you want to eat in the mall, but let's see how busy it is."

She huffed at me, and we headed in to get burritos. The lines were short in front of each restaurant, and she patiently waited her turn. You could hear the buzz of people talking throughout the food court, the smell of food being made, clanging of kitchen utensils and music playing overhead. I looked at her, and she was still holding her own, to my surprise. She proudly told the guy behind the counter what she wanted on her burrito before we paid and went to find a seat. As we moved through the seating, the music and talking was louder.

"Why don't we pick a booth? It will be quieter, and we will have our own space." We sat down, and she looked at me with a huge smile.

"Mommy, this is soooo cool! I am eating lunch at the mall!" Felicia bounced in her seat with a huge smile on her face.

I couldn't help but laugh at her excitement. This was a huge outing for her—and so far, she was doing it successfully. We ate and talked away. I watched her eyes wander up to the ceiling, looking at the lights that hung above us. She watched the people and now and then, her arms and legs would stim with excitement before she would go back to eating. When we were done, we decided to head to the bookstore. They had toys, and I thought we might as well take advantage of a successful outing and let her look around. We walked through the mall. She pointed at different stores and told me she should buy a wig for dress-up, because she would look "so amazing." When we got to the bookstore, she beelined it for the brightly-coloured baby toys, and I let her. She analyzed each one, pressing buttons and watching lights. I don't know how often you see a nine-year-old so content in the baby section. I tried to guide her into a different aisle to see if anything else would catch her eye, but she skimmed the aisles like she could care less. I thought some of the craft kits looked kind of interesting, but nope—she spotted the purple whale on a bath toy, and she was gone again, back to the baby aisle. I looked at the time, and it was time to hit the road.

"Come on, Felicia, time to go." Unlike years before when I would have to carry her kicking and screaming to the stroller, she calmly put down what she was looking at and took my hand, and we walked out. We headed back in the direction we came in and as we approached, the sounds of the food court hit us like a wall. *Why is it necessary to have the music so loud over here?* Felicia looked at me and I nodded. "We are almost there, just out the door." She picked up the pace—she now wanted out. We made it through the door and into the fresh air. We had done it. We had eaten lunch at the mall.

"Mommy, that was noisy, but that was like the best lunch *ever*." She skipped back to the truck.

When Ashley got home that night, she could not wait to tell her about her amazing time.

"Mom, I ate lunch at the mall. We ate in a boob because it was quieter."

"A boob? You mean a *booth*." Ashley looked at her, laughing.

"Yeah, Mom . . . a boob. That's what I said."

This time, we had done it. This time, it was successful. As a person who doesn't have sensory issues, I can filter the extra sensory input of the sounds, smells, and sights. Children and adults with autism and sensory processing disorder can't. It's like being hit with all your senses on high, all at once. Next time you are at the mall, I want you to sit in a booth and pay attention to everything you hear, see, and smell. Make yourself overly aware of everything around you. At the end of this book, I will provide a link where you can have a sensory experience that was created by a woman who has autism to give neurotypical people the opportunity to see the world in a different way.

The world isn't as accessible as you may think. Yes, we have many ramps, buttons to open doors, wheelchair- accessible parking—but have you ever tried to navigate a wheelchair through a store? Have you ever tried to grocery shop with a child who has mobility issues who is too big to fit in the cart?

Before Christmas, I had to stop at our local bulk store for some odds and ends. Chase was on a running streak—especially in public—when he got excited over things he loved. We parked and I loaded him into the stroller before we headed into the store. Our special-needs stroller is approximately the size of a regular wheelchair and turns on a dime. I absolutely love it. The stroller gives me the freedom to shop without worrying about Chase's safety and mobility.

I turned down one of the aisles, filling our bags with ingredients. I had promised the kids we would make sugar cookies. As I went to move to the next aisle, I couldn't get around the end display—there wasn't enough room for the stroller to fit between the bins and the display. The aisle was also too narrow, and I couldn't turn the stroller around. I walked backwards, all the way back up the aisle. I went to turn down the opposite end of the next aisle, and again, the stroller barely fit. I knocked off bags of chips off the bottom of the rack all over the floor. I parked the stroller and quickly ran down the next aisle, grabbed what I needed, and jogged back before Chase could touch anything else. I grabbed what I needed and made it to the cash register and paid. As we went to leave, I couldn't get the stroller between the boxes they had piled at the end of the cash. I had to pick the stroller up and position it perfectly before I could move forward. I still hit three boxes, and they toppled over as we went by and out the door.

I'd like to say that this is the only store we've run into problems with, but honestly, most of the stores—especially clothing stores, you cannot navigate with a stroller or wheelchair through safely. If I had been an adult in a wheelchair trying to pick up food for myself, this trip would have been even more of a nightmare. As Chase gets older I take note on where is accessible and where is not. Ableism is the discrimination in favour of able-bodied people. In this case, the store had been set up for able-bodied people. The bins were all set back for people who could stand and see inside. The aisles were not wide enough to be fully accessible, and there were hazards for anyone in a wheelchair or walker—or who had visual impairment—at every turn. Lack of accessibility is a form of ableism.

Chase is seven. He has long legs and weighs almost fifty pounds, which is getting heavy to lift in and out of anything—especially for myself, as I am only five foot three inches tall. His leg braces add to the weight, and his feet don't have the range of motion a child without leg braces has. Last week, I had to stop to get groceries. He wasn't having a great balance day—and he also loves to touch things on the store shelves. Imagine having a child, fast as lightening, but staggers around like your drunk friend at the bar who has had one too many. For his own safety, and the safety of every store display, he needs to be contained. However, taking his stroller isn't an option in grocery stores, as I have nowhere to put the groceries.

On this day, we parked beside the carts (everyone always tries to park near the door—pro tip: park beside the carts it always makes shopping with kids easier), and I grabbed a cart. I lifted him up to put him into the seat at the front, and I couldn't get him in. His shoes and his braces wouldn't fit through the holes anymore. I put him back down.

"OK, buddy, you have to sit in the big part, and mommy has to put the groceries in with you, OK? You cannot get out of the cart. You stay in the cart. Do you understand?"

He nodded, and I sat him in the lower section of the two-tiered cart. His legs barely fit, and he looked uncomfortable. We were going to get this done, we could do this. We headed into the store. A lady stared at us as we passed her, thinking, I'm sure, *why can't that kid walk?*

We wandered the produce aisle, and Chase pointed out all the fruits and vegetables as we went by. We headed to the grocery aisles, and I watched him get antsy as I started putting things into the cart around him. He was excited about the waffles we were getting, and crushed the boxed in between his hands. Next thing

I knew, he was trying to bring home all the granola bars off the shelf, reaching along the shelves, trying to add things to the cart as we went.

"Chase, don't touch. We don't need those." He was grabbing boxes faster than I could put them back on the shelf. When we are in public, I tend to use sign language and my voice. When my hands move, they catch his eye gaze, and I know he hears me. I grabbed his hands in mine and put my face up to his.

"Chase, look at me. Stop!" Telling Chase to stop was like telling someone to calm down—it didn't work. But I was watching his little body amp up, and I just needed him to breathe. "You stay in the cart. You don't touch." My time was limited, and I knew it. We were at the stage of get-in-and-get-out—whatever I missed, I would grab later.

We made it to the cash in one piece, and then Chase decided he was going to try to help put everything on the belt, since it was all around him and was easily accessible. As I started reaching to put things up, he started throwing boxes up onto the belt faster than I could grab them. Our groceries went every which way as they travelled towards the cashier. I grabbed the flat of eggs just as he was about to toss them up. The cashier looked at us and smiled as she scanned our upside-down milk, and I could feel myself starting to spiral from our own chaos. I sat the cart at the end of the cash and started to bag the groceries as fast as I could. As I packed our bags, they didn't fit the same way in the cart as they did before. I had to take Chase out of the cart to put them in. As he watched his favourite snacks get bagged, he would squeal in excitement and take them back out so he could look at the boxes. I grabbed his hand in mine and held it tight as I tried to pack the rest of our groceries and load them. Finally, I gave up, and tossed all the groceries, loose, back in the cart. I would bag them at the truck. I paid, and held his hands on the cart handle, and got him to help me push the heavy cart back to the parking lot, holding tight to keep him safe and from running when he saw our truck. I loaded him back into his car seat, did up his five-point harness, and went back to bagging my groceries beside the truck in the pouring rain.

We are constantly encouraged to take our children into the public. To teach them life skills, such as shopping. Yet everywhere we go, we hit roadblocks that make it near-impossible to focus on what we need to, because we are too busy focusing on how to navigate the world that isn't made accessible. A woman in the US named Drew Ann Long designed a shopping cart so she could take her growing daughter with disabilities and toddler grocery-shopping. She called it "Caroline's Cart," after her daughter. It is designed for your child, an adult with a disability, or a senior to sit in an actual, full seat in front of you, complete with safety belts—and it has a full cart for your groceries. Why aren't they everywhere? Why did a special-needs parents have to design and create this only recently, when there have been parents and seniors struggling for decades?

As my son gets older, we must also think about how to take him into bathrooms in public. If there is no family bathroom, then we must take him into a women's bathroom. Many women do not take kindly to a young man being taken into a women's bathroom. However, I cannot send him alone into the men's bathroom, as he is not only a vulnerable person, but he might also need assistance—and I can't do that from the hallway. Parents who have children who require incontinence products often don't find change tables that are large enough for their children, leaving them to change their older children and teenagers on the dirty bathroom floor. Children and adults with disabilities deserve to be treated with dignity, regardless of their diagnosis or physical capability. Lying on a bathroom floor does not do that.

The Oxford Dictionary uses this definition for the word inclusion: *the practice, or policy of providing equal access to opportunities and resources for people who might otherwise be excluded or marginalized, such as those who have physical or mental disabilities and members of other minority groups.*

To create a truly inclusive world, people need to be given accessibility to be independent. To be able to grocery shop in a safe accessible space. To be able to go to a store with a wheelchair and try on clothes. I know plenty of young adults who want to have all the same experiences as their peers, like shopping and hanging out with their friends at a mall. But the stores they want to go into are not accessible for wheelchairs, walkers, or for someone with visual impairment. Obstacles litter the walking path, and the aisles are not wide enough to navigate.

As a society, we can do better—but it needs to be more than special-needs parents fighting for change. We need society to see where we are falling short for our neighbours, friends, and family, and start to make changes.

The opportunities that our children will have in the future are ones that we create by surrounding ourselves with like-minded people wanting the same change. Change can happen with something as simple as "sensory hours" at a local entertainment venue. It can be accessible shopping carts at the grocery store. It can be creating a special-needs program within a community program. It can be making sure a wheelchair can get through the aisles of a store, and it can be educating the people around us about what challenges our families face, so that other people want to see change as well. I know every new age will come with new roadblocks we will be facing as a family, but the more we bring awareness about inclusion and accessibility to people in our lives, the more we will start seeing things change in the world around us.

TWENTY-TWO: Connections

Human connection—isn't that something we all strive for? To be able to say, I have a family who loves me, friends who share common interests with me, or a group of people with shared experiences I can connect with. Human connection is a basic need that we strive to have met. That's why everyone is searching for approval on social media isn't it?

Society looks at people with autism and they only see a person keeping to themselves—a child, anxious and doing repetitive behaviours, hand-flapping and talking to themselves. They see behaviours, and children chewing on chewlry, or wearing noise cancelling headphones. They see the weird kid. When instead, we should be looking at each person as an individual with interests, thoughts and opinions. Such as Adam, the little boy who loves everything that involves recycling. Anne, who loves reading books about the best playwrights in history, or Skylar, who loves all things Disney. They want to talk to people about their interests, to engage, and to feel seen. A lack of human connection through friendships and love has a massive impact on our overall health. Mental health challenges and feelings of loneliness are exceptionally high among people on the spectrum. Even though an autistic person may look like they want to keep to themselves, they are often the ones who need the opportunity for connection the most.

Think back to when the world stopped during the start of the pandemic in 2020. How many people felt isolated and lonely? How many people wanted to connect with family and friends, and couldn't? What did that do to your mental health? Now, imagine if that was how you lived all the time. Many people with disabilities often do.

Ever since Chase was little, he has sought out all forms of human connection. He loves to be in the middle of everything, even when he really shouldn't be. If you're cooking, he wants to be sitting on the counter, watching. If you are building something, he brings his toys over, so he is with you. When Ashley works on the Jeep in the driveway, he has his cars outside, sitting beside her. Before he had any verbal communication, he would use any form he could to make sure you knew what he wanted. Between the speech he has and his speech device, he will make sure you know what he wants—and if I don't acknowledge him right away, all I hear is "Mommy, Mommy, Mommy . . .", and he will get right into my face, with his little finger pointed at my eyeball, so I pay attention to him. People always assume he can't answer questions due to his limited speech, and they will ask me to answer for him.

"Does Chase want an apple for a snack?"

I look at them and then at him. "Ask him . . . ."

Just because a child or adult with disabilities cannot speak doesn't mean they don't have opinions about what they like or don't like, and about the world around them.

I used to tell my volunteers at the barn during lessons, "Just because the riders don't respond doesn't mean they can't hear you. Look them in the eye and talk to them. It's basic human connection. If you're rider is an adult, do not baby-talk them. Talk to them as you would any other adult—they are all people who need to be treated with dignity."

Chase has a decent level of stranger-danger, but once he gets to know you, he is all over you. Except therapists—they must earn his full trust before he will work for them. He loves our family—especially his grandparents—as most kids do. However, my dad, his Papa, is the holy grail of people in his life. If Papa is around, the rest of us are ghosts in his little world. It's a relationship I always wanted for him. A connection with someone that was just his. He tells me when he's big he will drive the boat like Papa does. I tell him we will make sure he does.

When Felicia was little, she was more about surface relationships. She wanted the attention, but letting people in—well, that was a different story. She knew who she could manipulate into doing things she wanted. She would cling to grandparents when Ashley and I would ask her to do things just so she didn't have to. She is a master at reading people, and seeing their weaknesses and strengths. It has always been impressive to witness. The only person she didn't seem to play off of was Ashley's grandpa.

As you've come to know, the early years were hard. She was stuck in her own ball of chaos. But around him, she would just . . . be. We would go over to Ashley's mother's house, where her grandparents also lived, and Felicia would disappear into the basement. We would find her sitting with her Great Pa in his recliner, almost eighty years apart in age, but content to be together. His hearing wasn't the best, and she had a speech delay. I don't think either of them knew what each other was ever saying, but they had their own language, which none of us really understood. She would stand and brush his hair for him, or sit on his bed and play with a singing fish he had. More than often, she would be sitting with him watching the weather network and God only knows what else with him—but they were happy, and we didn't intervene. He had been ill for a while, and we knew his time was limited. We were all aware of how close Felicia had become to him, and how much loss she had already experienced in her life.

Only the Strong Survive

But we watched this little girl who was struggling so much finally just be content—and he loved her so much. Why deprive either of them of that special kind of bond?

In the summer, the backyard would be filled with birdfeeders, and it came to life from his flowers he wanted planted. He would feed the squirrels, and he would sit in his walker, cracking peanuts open for Felicia to eat. For his birthday, Felicia wanted to make him a new birdhouse. So, we went to the store and picked up a kit. She sat at our dining room table, meticulously painted it, and then insisted on wrapping it by herself. It was the first time she showed any interest in giving anyone a gift—let alone making them something. But this was her Great Pa, and she would do anything for him. On his birthday, she proudly stood in front of him and handed over his gift. He looked at her with a big smile on his face, and opened it, inspecting her paint job. He made sure it was hung front and centre in the garden.

A few years passed, and he began getting sicker—and we knew the time was coming, and we tried to prepare her the best we could. The day he passed away, I called her to the dining room table.

"Felicia, honey, we need to have a talk." I didn't have to go any further. She knew . . . .

"Did Great Pa pass away?"

I nodded, and for the first time ever, I watched this little girl fall apart not from rage, not from a meltdown, but from pure, raw emotion. I held her tight while she sobbed in my arms. I was at peace with him passing, but I cried for my daughter and all that she had lost.

A few days later, she looked at me and asked, "But what is happening to Great Pa's things? They aren't going in the garbage, right?"

"No. No, we aren't going to throw away Great Pa's things. We will give them to people in the family and to people who need

them—but nothing is going in the garbage. Would you like to go over and see if there is something you would like to keep?"
She nodded.
I looked at Ashley that night and shook my head. "You know what she's going to want to bring home, right?"
"Uh-huh—and I have no idea how we are going to fit it in the house. We have nowhere to put it."
"We can rearrange her room, maybe?" We would have to figure something out.
We headed over to Ashley's mom's the next day, and went down into his room. Felicia looked around, missing her best friend.
"OK, Felicia you can pick anything you want to have so you can remember Great Pa."
And just like we had predicted, she lifted her finger and pointed. "I want his chair . . . ."
Ashley and I looked at each other, and then at the well-worn, old, blue recliner. The one they had spent hours in together. The one they had told stories in, and she brushed had his hair in.
"OK." Ashley's mom would get it cleaned, and then we would pick it up.
That old blue chair now sits in her bedroom, and I often find her curled up in it while she plays on her iPad. It is her comfort spot. Everyone has questioned how a man so sick was able to live years past his diagnosed life expectancy. I think some of those years were reserved for Felicia, and I am so happy that they were. Despite the greatness of the loss, Felicia got to experience the greatness of the connection and love that she will carry with her forever.
A few weeks after his passing, Felicia looked at us and asked about what happens after you die. In our house, autism is black and white, without room for grey. Thoughts and ideas must be clear and direct. I once made the mistake of saying "this carwash is taking forever" while in the line-up for the carwash. She burst

into a mass hysteria in the backseat. She thought the car wash was literally taking forever. All her hopes and dreams were about to be washed away. For months, we couldn't even pass that area without her cursing out the carwash. You know how many random figures of speech we use every day? I didn't either—until Felicia.

So, when it came to death, I had tried the scientific approach — the very clean-cut, when-you-die-your-body-turns-to-dirt approach—but she wasn't having it. I am not a religious person, so I wasn't going down the heaven-and-hell road with her—and that is way to abstract for discussion. We went back and forth about how to handle the talk about death again. When she was little and we had lost animals, she had just accepted that they were gone. But with her favourite person in the whole wide world, that wasn't going to be the case.

Ashley sat her down one day after she asked again, and without missing a beat she said, "Great Pa went to a super cool place." Felicia was now intrigued. "You can only go there when you pass away, though. You have to live your whole life first, and get super old."

"Does it have ice cream?" Her eyes widened with the thought.

"Absolutely!"

"Can I play with Great Pa?"

"Yes, you can, all you want."

"Can Great Pa roll down the hill and do somersaults with me?" She giggled with excitement at the thought of her Great Pa rolling down a hill—her arms and legs were stimming now.

"Yep, he can. His body isn't sick anymore there, and he can do anything he wants." Well, that was it . . . when she died, she could go to the "super cool place" where they have endless ice cream and she and Great Pa can run, jump, and play. She came up with grand ideas after that about what else could be done in the "super cool place," and we let her. She was able to cope with the idea that people leave us, but she would get to see them again. Sometimes, our methods don't always make sense—but they work.

Today, Felicia is a nine-year-old, fighting for independence, as little girls do. She wants to be a "big girl," she tells me. Parts of her brain are ready, and in other parts, she's still little, and naïve to the scary world that is around her. She decided to take herself for a walk by herself around the block a couple weeks ago without telling anyone, and once we found her, we gave her a that's-not-safe, we-don't-just-leave-the-driveway talk.

She looked at us and said, "I just went for a walk, and I was talking to the neighbours."

My heart sank. She had zero sense of stranger-danger. We had been working on this for years, and it was not sinking in.

"It's not safe talking to strangers, Felicia. you don't know who is good and who is bad in the world. We want to keep you safe. You don't talk to people you don't know . . ."

And as I continued with my spiel, she looked at me so innocently, and said, "I was just trying to put positive into the world, not negative."

That was it. I was done.

My whole body dropped, and I fought back tears . . . . I nodded. "I know, honey . . . ."

This little girl was trying so hard to navigate the social world, and trying so hard to fit in.

My children show us every day that they strive for connections. They want to love and be loved. They want to fit into a world that is not quite made for them, and have human connections, just like everyone else. Every time a person talks *around* a person with a disability and not *to* them, or doesn't ask about their opinions, thoughts, and dreams, or doesn't provide them inclusion and opportunity to participate, they are denying them of basic connections that help them thrive. Even when someone is not avoided but given a simple smile and hello can make all the difference in the world.

TWENTY-THREE:
Into the Forest I Go . . .

"Into the forest I go, to lose myself and find my soul."—John Muir

It's hard being everything for everyone. We do so many tasks in a week sometimes, they just all blend together—and you lose yourself in routines, parenting, chores. But when was the last time you did something all by yourself, for longer than a day? I don't mean that glorious alone grocery-shopping trip, or finally going to the dentist . . . something you *wanted* to do.

Last summer, I went on vacation by myself, to the woods, alone, for five days. Sounds crazy, right? What made me go into the scary woods, alone, with potential serial killers lurking behind every bush, you ask? After five years of parenting two high-demand kids, I could actually feel my soul trying to physically leave my body—to escape to somewhere different. I was claustrophobic the moment my eyes opened in the morning. It took every ounce of me to get out of bed in the morning and get things done—even the things I enjoyed felt like a chore. I felt like I was buried ten feet down, and couldn't resurface—and I had never felt like this in my life. I was willing to greet the serial killers in the woods with open arms.

I've never vacationed anywhere alone—let alone somewhere off the grid—but I decided that I needed to be uncomfortable. I needed to prove to myself I could still do things that were out of the norm for me, that I could live beyond the walls of our home. They may call this a "mom crisis"—it's like a midlife crisis, but for moms. My bag was packed three days before I was going to leave. I was ready. And on the day of, I kissed my wife and kids goodbye and left. I don't even think I waved. I drove two hours, with my favourite music blaring, an hour and a half away from our home. It was a tiny home on someone's property in their woods. They had one campsite on one side, and on another campsite, a shipping container home. I knew from the listing it had enough electricity to plug in my phone, no running water, an outdoor shower, a toilet, a BBQ, and silence.

I pulled up, and the owner met me in the driveway. He explained how I had to follow the woodchip path over the small wooden bridge, and then I'd be at the site. So, I unloaded my truck into a wagon, trying to stuff as many things as I could, hoping to only do one trip. I'm a one-trip kind of girl. You should see me bring in the groceries. If there was an Olympic event for it, I would win. And off I went into the woods, with my art supplies in hand.

I stumbled through the woods. The "bridge" was not a bridge, for the record—it was three planks of wood just big enough for the wagon to fit on, with less than an inch to spare on either side. In that moment, I had a flashback to me holding up the double stroller, knee-deep in the creek, so I creeped along very slowly—probably slower than I needed to—then, finally, in the clearing, was the tiny home. It was cute and well put together. My home for the next five days.

I unpacked—which, when you are not travelling with children, takes, like, no time at all, and makes you second-guess if you have everything. It was too early for dinner, so I sat down in silence—just me and the trees, I looked around and went, "What the fuck am I doing?" I literally said it out loud. It wasn't like anyone was around to hear me. I felt uncomfortable in the silence, my body and mind could not relax. I got up and went into the tiny home, seeing what I could find to cook with.

My family and I spent our summers at the cottage during my childhood, and it was what my dad called "a true cottage." We had limited electricity. We had a tiny bathroom, but the outhouse was much more reliable. We spent our summers in the lake, by the fire, slathered in sunscreen. You were taught how to drive the boat at the age of twelve, and we would go worm-hunting in the back field at night with flashlights, so we could fish off the dock.

Eventually, I had to give into the fact that I had to go to the bathroom, so I headed to the back of the site to find the outdoor toilet. I was instantly taken back to my childhood—except this outdoor toilet had no walls like the one I grew up with. It was a Thunderbox—a wooden box with a lid—and when you opened it, there was a hole to sit on, and your toilet paper and hand sanitizer in a Ziplock bag, so the bugs didn't get in. Even when you know you no one is around you, still feel insanely exposed sitting on that toilet, just you and the trees and the birds and the bugs. There was no way in hell I was going to stumble to the back of the campsite in the dark, with mosquitos, to use this thing. Liquids would be limited before bed, and my last trip would be planned right before dark. If serial killers were going to get me, it sure as hell wouldn't be sitting on the Thunderbox.

When you are from a decent-sized city, you forget just how dark the nights can be—especially with a treetop canopy. The bed in the tiny home was in the loft section. You had to climb this very steep staircase/ladder. It was just tall enough that I could sit on the floor and my head would be touching the ceiling. When I laid on the bed, I had to make sure I didn't sit up too quickly, or I would whack my forehead on the planked ceiling. I tucked myself in way earlier than normal. I had downloaded a few shows into my iPad to watch at night to wind down, and then, I settled to try to get some sleep. It had been big day. Nature is not quiet at night, and there were many sounds that I had no idea what they were. Keep in mind: we cottaged, we did not tent-camp growing up. I don't ever remember nature being that loud. Being alone in the forest reminds you of how many fun scenarios your brain can come up with, *and would anyone find the body?* It took forever to fall asleep.

I woke up the next morning—still alive, might I add—and realized I didn't have to get out of bed if I didn't want to. I laid there for a while. There was no one to make breakfast for, no one needing anything. I could do whatever I wanted in my own time, without expectation. The morning was cold compared to the night before, and I was restless. I made my way down the loft ladder and found the coffee, the jug of water, and the matches. This, I knew how to do—lighting a burner and cooking off a propane stove—I had skills I had forgotten about.

I gave up on the French press pretty quickly and opted for the small coffee filters, and steeped my coffee grounds by hand. When you've got time, these small things don't seem so annoying—where did I have to rush to anyway? I came to enjoy that process every morning. It felt intentional. I read a blog once about how you should take the time to focus on one thing at a time to bring joy back into that one task, so I was going to try it. I took my coffee outside and sat in a blue Adirondack chair. Today, I was going to drink my coffee in nature, and not do anything else until it was done. The urge to multitask was insane—like I couldn't settle my brain into *just being*.

I became aware very quickly on how much I moved in a day, never stopping. I had to force myself to do such a simple task—sit and drink coffee—and I was sad for myself in that moment. I took a deep breath and closed my eyes, trying to find the sounds of the forest instead of the voice inside of my head. The first day was dedicated to slowing down, eating a meal, and focusing on *just* the meal, picking up my art supplies and working away, reading only

Only the Strong Survive

a chapter of my book at a time, taking it in slowly .... It wasn't easy, but the more I focused on living with intention, the more I could feel myself relax and started enjoying being in the moment.

Since December, I had been battling breathing issues and a chronic cough from a post-viral infection, and was going through testing and testing medications, without success. The humid weather made breathing harder, and the summer was proving to be a challenge already. As I finally let my shoulders relax without added stress, my cough wasn't as bad, I could breathe outside for the first time in months. I realized the pressure I was putting on myself was making me sicker. If this was going to be a chronic illness, I needed to learn how to pace myself—to live it with it and stop fighting. Were things really working the old way anyway? Clearly not.

The outdoor shower was my greatest love-hate relationship that week. Outdoor showers have a limited water supply, so you get wet, turn it off, soap up, turn it on . . . it's this back-and-forth dance. Though it was hot back home—like, that sticky, can't-sit-outside hot—it was just comfortable in the woods. As the sun peered through the trees, I would move my chair around in the sunspots it made on the woodchip ground to suntan. The outdoor shower, however, was not in a sunspot—therefore, the water in the barrel was only heated by the air temperature, and the nights would cool down, and so would the barrel. The first day I stepped into the wooden box and flicked on that water, I gasped, trying to catch my breath in the freezing water. I am a person who likes hot showers—I mean scalding-your-skin hot, until the shower runs cold—it is my Zen before I start my day. This was an experience that would test my willpower for cleanliness. I started to try to figure out ways of how to avoid the shower, but, in the end, my need to feel clean and get the layers of bug spray off always won. There was no way in hell I was going to shave my legs in there. A bowl of water I left in the sun, though . . . now *that* I could work with. I sat in the sun and got nice and hot before running to the shower get clean, then dry back in the sun. I had a method.

When you are completely alone, you don't talk . . . like, at all. I didn't use my voice for days, which is a weird concept considering how much I repeated myself in a day—because let's be honest: kids don't listen. When was the last time you didn't say a word for a full day to anyone? When the kids called me a few days into my trip, my voice sounded almost foreign. I thought about calling home for bedtimes, but that would defeat the purpose of this trip, and I was afraid if I talked to home I would get sucked into the busy again. But I knew with my children's attachment insecurities, they needed to know I was there when they needed me. We chatted for a few minutes, and when I hung up the phone, I was able to tell myself there was nothing I could do at home, and went back to my book.

I wear a lot of hats, for a lot of people and animals, to the point that some weeks, I can't keep up . . . . I'm an appointment-scheduler, a play-the-role occupational therapist, physiotherapist, speech therapist, behaviour therapist, I'm an acting dietician and researcher—hell, with my credentials if I wanted to work, no one could afford me. I am a wife, a mom, an aunt, a daughter . . . for me, I'm an artist and a horse mom . . . . And each of these things take pieces of me that are no longer mine.

During this process, I realized the parts of me that had been buried long before children—like how much I love nature, how much I love reading. I can use propane stoves, start fires—and I'm not scared of outdoor toilets, like one might assume. I love looking at the textures of nature—such as tree bark, leaves, water—how they all play off each other and contrast yet complement one another. It inspires me artistically. I crave water and being around any body of it—and there was none around me on this trip, and I could feel myself twitch. I wondered what else had I been missing in my life.

By the last night, I was ready to be done. It took everything not to run out of those woods and not look back. I promised myself

I was going to finish this journey, and *damnit*, I was. So, instead, I packed everything I could that night, and in the morning, I was out two hours before checkout time. I took one last look at that tiny home before I made it back around the plank bridge and I said thank you. As much as I was ready, I was sad to leave that ultimate feeling of peace I felt behind.

I felt like I had recharged for the first time in years—like I could handle the meltdowns and constant pull again. I felt level-headed and at ease. I felt like a version of myself I hadn't recognized in a long time. Before I would head home to our everyday chaos, I headed to the beach for the day.

I must have given off a relaxed vibe at the beach. I have never had so many random locals come up and sit and talk with me before. It was like I had a sign pointing over me: "Over here—free small talk!" I was there long enough to see Gladys have her first swim of the day and then come back for her afternoon swim later. She had arthritis, you know, and if she doesn't have her two swims a day, it acted up in the summer. I couldn't help but chuckle. I hope to be like Gladys when I grow up.

On my way home, I stopped off at the local winery for some of my favourite wine, then ended my day with the longest, hottest shower and I will never take that luxury for granted again. It was followed by the sound of my family coming through the front door for everyday life to start up again.

I will make a conscious effort to do this again. For me to be able to be everything I need to be for everyone else, I need to be a whole person. Would I suggest trying something like this to someone else? Absolutely! You don't have to be in the woods, but extended time alone, on your terms, is good for the soul. Flight attendants tell us to put our oxygen masks on before helping someone else for a reason, and that applies to all aspects of our lives. Next time, though, I will bring more than one book—and I will try to be closer to water.

TWENTY-FOUR:
The Future

"Your children won't be with you forever . . . ." I've heard this from so many people in the last few years—almost like they haven't listened to anything we have said about the reality of our children's disabilities, or they refuse to accept the answer because they have a hard time with realistic hope.

From day one, when the kids came home, our goal has always been to give them as many skills as possible, to make them as independent as we possibly can, in hopes they can grow into productive people in society. Even if they can't work, they can volunteer their time and give back in some way.

When we think long term, our reality is prepping for every scenario, and trying to stick with realistic hopes and goals. Our kids are little, and I understand that we have a long way to go (believe me, we work beyond hard for every advancement).

Things we know, though, are that Chase has limited speech, it is unknown if people will be able to understand him, and he may need his speech device for the rest of his life. My children will not legally be allowed to drive a car—but independent bus transportation is an obtainable goal. I do not believe either child will be able to live on their own or have a family of their own. We will try to teach skills that may be able to help them maybe find a small, part-time job.

We prepare and focus on skills that are important for everyday living—making their own food, paying for things with money, cleaning the house, learning how to have appropriate conversations and communicate their needs. We also worry if will they have the skills to be independent once we are gone, and we worry about what happens if they don't. Will there be suitable housing and services for them? Could we afford those services for the rest of their lives? I hope society grows with us, but without getting political, I am fearful of that, too—and how do I prepare for the lack of resources available to disabled adults? It's almost all too big to think about all at once—it's easier to focus on the day to day.

Every parent worries about their children's future—it comes with the job. We can all worry, for so many different reasons—disabilities involved or not. But when people state, "Ah, your kids won't be with you forever, so cherish them now . . .", sometimes I smile and nod, and other times, if I have the energy, I educate on what it's like to have a child with a disability and the reality of what the future *really* looks like.

The truth is nobody can tell us what will happen in the future. Like every other special-needs parent, you pray you live forever so you never have to worry about what will happen to your children after you are gone.

Ashley and I are trying hard to put things in place now so that we can grow into the next stage of our lives with our children, and push for as much independence as we can. Part of that plan is a bigger house with an in-law suite potential, with accessibility—so no matter what happens with Chase's cerebellar hypoplasia, he will be able to navigate his space safely. We will continue with programs wherever their interests lie, keeping them active and social. We hope for strong family bonds and making memories with Nana, Papa, Grandma, aunts, uncles, and cousins.

Felica has come a long way since laying in puddles. Her big new goal is turning sixteen. When Felicia was around the age of four, she decided to replace all numbers when counting with the word "fucker." I wish I was lying. We would be sitting on the floor, and she would be building a tower with blocks, and we would be trying to encourage her to count "one, two, three . . .", and she would go "fucker, fucker, fucker . . . ." Having to explain that one to people was not a proud parenting moment. We had to tell her that she was too little to use bad words, and she came back with, "Well, how old do I have to be?" On a whim Ashley told her she could had to be sixteen . . . *thanks, Ash*. So now, she proudly tells people when she's sixteen she's allowed to say bad words—and she will hold us to it. We've got six years left to keep the cap on that. I'd like to say we are rocking this parenting thing, but I'm not so sure.

I have learned over the years that Felicia is like the sun. People gravitate toward her. Sometimes, she burns them, but it doesn't stop them from coming back for more—because sometimes, that sunshine doesn't burn, but it glows bright and warm, and is so inviting. The people who surround her see her potential and want her to succeed to her fullest. They want to be a part of her story. We gravitated to her, didn't we? As we move into the preteen years, we will be in for a whole other level of unknown territory. I'm not ready for puberty, and will take all the help I can get from our support system around us. I will also start taking wine donations now.

Public school has been our newest adventure. She loves school and taking the bus. She loves gymnastics, biking, and swimming as if she was born in the water. She loves to help around the barn with the horses, and you can't tell her that the wheelbarrow is too heavy to push—she's determined and stubborn, and will prove you wrong every time. Felicia is a movie junkie—if it's a kid movie, she has seen it. She often asks if she can watch a movie she's never seen. We are struggling to find new ones at this point. Soon, she will be counting down the days it will be warm enough to be back at the beach, and all will be right in her world. Until then, she's jumping in puddles and asking if she can play in the rain. She will be ten this year. I'd love to take her to a waterpark. Her eyes light up with excitement at the thought of waterslides, and a whole park made up of her favourite thing in the world—not to mention staying in a hotel for the first time. We will see if we can make it happen. If she wants to try, then I want to try my best to make it happen.

Chase is in full little-boy mode. We still work hard with therapy every week. He's trying hard to say three-word sentences. He now has an augmentative and alternate communication device (AAC), or, as we call it, his "talker." It is an iPad with a speech device app on it. It's filled with pictures and words, and he can tap on the words and make full sentences. He uses it to ask for things he wants, communicate his needs, or just have a conversation. It has opened his entire world, and it's confirming just how smart we always knew he was. He is creative, and loves to be a jokester. I often say he's the perfect little brother—he knows exactly how to get under his sister's skin, and finds true joy in making her scream over silly things. He loves Mickey Mouse, *Teenage Mutant Ninja Turtles*, and *RuPaul's Drag Race*. I am pretty sure his life goal is to be a drag queen. He wants to wear fancy dresses for dress-up and have "big pink hair," he tells me. He's got the moves. If we just work on his make-up application, he might just do it. If he's happy, then I am happy.

He's recently formed a tight bond with our new rescue horse, which took me off guard. He's never been one to gravitate towards animals, but this thousand-pound black horse stole his heart. I am fairly sure he's the size of Theo's head, but they are besties, who wear matching outfits—including hats with pom-poms. That horse is an absolute saint.

For a child who took so long to walk, and still falls often, he moves at the speed of light, never walking. When it was time to be discharged from the therapy centre, I cried after every session in the truck for a month before we were done. The thought of losing our team was too much to bear. They had been my support system for almost four years. They watched him grow, change, and overcome obstacles. Anytime we run into them, they watch him in amazement—some even fight back tears—and it confirms our hard work is paying off. Chase and I had tried another private therapist, but it just wasn't a good fit. His old occupational therapist decided to go into private services, and I jumped on the opportunity. We had to start therapy via Zoom, but the moment that screen turned on, it instantly felt like we were coming home. We are still trying to figure out what the best learning option is for him. Nothing seems to feel like a good fit, and I worry about this ability to advocate for himself, due to his communication barriers—or to tell us if something is not right. He is still home with me, and I am doing the best I can to build a solid foundation for him. We are thinking about trying a private special-needs school. New adventures and challenges await.

Ashley and I are finally back to being the dream team. It took a while. It felt like we were living on two different islands for a while—or like roommates who pass each other in the hall and sit down for a meal now and then. We both had things to work through, and it is not easy—especially while raising children. We are on the same path for our future again. We sit down and "conference" regularly on what we need to do for the kids, and what is working and what is not. Special-needs parenting requires flexibility, and that's not always easy—for me, at least. Sometimes, I don't know how we've survived. There are times I didn't think we would—but then I look at her, and I don't know if I could do this journey with anyone else—or if I would want to. Are we still on the wild ride of marriage and parenting? Absolutely. Is it easy? Hell to the no.

Have you ever played the "if you could talk to your younger self" game with your spouse? We did a while back. It was after a hard, exhausting day of parenting. It had been one of those "why did we choose this path?" days. Ashley said she would go back and warn herself to stop while she was ahead.

"You have it so good, you don't know how good you have it. And I would shake the shit out of myself."

I laughed. "You really think our younger selves would have listened?"

We both shook our heads. We knew it wouldn't have worked. It would've just made us push on harder, and still would be where we are today. There are times we do think, *why did we do this?* I honestly believe there was a driving force pushing us in this direction. I don't think we really had any control. I haven't figured out why we are on this journey, but it's bigger than us—and one day, we will have that "ah-ha" moment and understand.

Just over a year ago, I looked at Ashley and said, "You know, I could see us adopting or fostering a teenager when we are older and more settled . . . ." I braced for the "are you nuts?" speech, but to my surprise, she didn't hate the idea. Teens are one of the hardest age categories to get adopted in the foster care system—especially if they are LGBTQ+. Many never find their families, and then age out, without ever having a solid home base and support system to come back to. Everyone wants to have a family cheering them on when they succeed, and a place they can call home when things get tough.

I should have known what happens when you throw these things out into the universe. Only days later, our teenage nephew messaged me: "Can I come?" And like that, he was on a plane . . . . His story is not mine to tell, so I will leave those details to him to share, but I can tell you navigating the teenage years is a whole other ballgame. He's thriving, though, and we are proud of him and all he's accomplishing. Ashley looked at me, shaking her head . . . . "We put it out there . . . ." I couldn't help but laugh. Apparently, the universe thought we were ready now, and that our plans were merely a suggestion in the grand scheme. I am learning how to go with the flow. Some days, that's easier said than done.

For me, my goals have changed. I have spent more time remembering I am a person, too, and I have things I need to do for myself. I am an artist (it took me a long time to say that)—I channel my energy and feelings into my paintings and then send them out into the world. Each piece of work is part of your soul being put on display. It's nerve wracking, but it makes you feel that spark of joy when it ends up on someone else's wall, and that your work and vision has touched them in some way.

I am an advocate, and I wear that title with pride. I advocate for my children, our family, and other families going through similar experiences, trying to navigate systems. Over the years, I have taken note of the resources parents lack—and I want to change that. In fact, it's my goal to change that. Whether it's getting onto the board at the children's centre or fighting for my children's needs in programs—in the school system or everyday life—advocacy never ends.

A few years ago, I came across a video that opened my world. It was a mom like me, talking about "the hard." It came at a time I was drowning, and it became so apparent how we don't share the honest struggles of not only parenting, but special-needs parenting. We hold our struggles close, head down, and move through life pretending like we are OK, and that we fit into boxes we clearly don't. Recently, I started a parent support group for local parents who needed to talk about "the hard." I knew how lonely it could be, and I knew other parents were out there struggling as well. Why were we all shuffling through alone when we could be together?

Only the Strong Survive

So much pressure is put on the early years of your child's life. You hear the sentences, "If we don't get ahead of this now . . .", "Children learn and change the most in the first five years . . .", "Early intervention is key . . .", and parents then stress about all the time they have left before the window closes. I agree early intervention is key for therapies—but for me, the stress of "missing the window of learning" has passed. We focus on stage versus age now. As humans, we are lifelong learners. Why are we trying to jam-pack it all into the early years? I will never give up on progression—but my kids have taught me that they will do it in their time, not ours. What I will continue to fight for is their future, though. Just like any other child, they deserve quality education, quality resources, and the opportunities to be included and experience all that life has to offer.

We didn't get to where we are by mistake. It has been years of grit, blood, sweat, and tears. Crumbling to the depths and rebuilding who we are. If you are in "the hard" right now, whether it be infertility, adoption, or parenting, I want you to know that even though it can feel so insanely isolating, you are not alone. There is someone out there who understands—and I, too, have been beaten down. I have been isolated. I have gotten to the point where I didn't think we'd see the light again. Sometimes, we can't find our community—we have to build it. We are all survivors in our own right. You will get through this. You will change and turn into the person you were supposed to be all along. You are meant for something bigger than your grief.

The tattoo that sits on my arm has gotten me this far. It is my self-boosting motto that reminds me I can get through anything. *Only the strong survive.* As a family, though, Ashley and I are stronger together—and we know that our two parts make a whole. Our family has come a long way, and the more we figure it all out together, the more I am convinced that we will make it—because the strong do not just survive, *the strong thrive.*

POST-ADOPTION DEPRESSION RESOURCES

www.adopt4life.com

https://www.adopt4life.com/adoption101-pads-post-adoption-depression

Adoption.com, "Post-Adoption Depression"

http://adopting.org/post-adoption-depression/

Adopting.com, "I Didn't Love My Child at First Sight"

http://adopting.org/i-didnt-love-my-child-at-first-sight/

"Symptoms of Post-Adoption Depression"

http://www.news-medical.net/health/Symptoms-of-Post-Adoption-Depression.aspx

Adoptive Families Association of BC, "Recognizing and Coping with Post-Adoption Depression"

https://www.bcadoption.com/resources/articles/recognizing-and-coping-post-adoption-depression

Adoptions Together, "Recognizing Post-Adoption Depression Syndrome"

https://www.adoptionstogether.org/blog/2013/01/07/why-arent-i-happy-recognizing-post-adoption-depression-syndrome/

Good Therapy, "Post-Adoption Depression in Fathers'"

http://www.goodtherapy.org/blog/fathers-post-adoption-depression-1110111/

Huffington Post, "What You Should Know About Post-Adoption Depression"

http://www.huffingtonpost.com/jill-robbins/what-you-should-know-abou_7_b_7985630.html

The Globe and Mail, "Post-Adoption Depression: A Condition Hard to Understand"

https://www.theglobeandmail.com/life/parenting/a-condition-hard-to-understand-post-adoption-depression/article4266093/

News Medical, "Contributing Factors to Post-Adoption Depression"

http://www.news-medical.net/health/Contributing-Factors-to-Post-Adoption-Depression.aspx

Adoption Council of Canada, "Post-Adoption Toolkit"

http://www.adoption.ca/uploads/File/ACC_Post-Adoption_Toolkit_Part2.pdf

She Knows, "The Reality of Post-Adoption Depression"

Ashley Biddiscombe

http://www.sheknows.com/parenting/articles/1002673/post-adoption-depression

Books

Karen J. Foli and John R. Thompson, *The Post-Adoption Blues: Overcoming the Unforeseen Challenges of Adoption.*

A Sensory Experience

https://www.carlyscafe.com/index_nf.html

ACKNOWLEDGEMENTS

There have been so many people along our journey that I need to thank.

First, to Angela, who has put more time and energy into our family than I can even express: your dedication to making sure that we made it, and continuing to support our family well after the adoption papers had been signed. We couldn't be where we are today without you.

To Melissa, you are one of the most amazing, strong, and inspiring women I have ever met. My children wouldn't be who they are today if you hadn't had the compassion and strength when they were starting of their lives. You've shown me the lengths that compassion can go to for birth parents, and just how amazing and dedicated foster parents can be.

To the therapist team that became an extension of our family—Carolyn, Heather, Sara, and Matthew and now Jenn—you saw us through some of our darkest days and you kept us going. Chase would not be where he is today without your dedicated support. He said his first words, took his first steps, did his first set of stairs in your care. On the days that were tough, you pushed to keep going. On the days we succeeded, you were there to cheer us on. Heather, I cannot thank you enough for being my sounding board, listening to my fears and not judging my tears.

Ashley Biddiscombe

To our respite workers, coaches, and teachers—Becca, Danielle, Shelley, Asifa, Laura . . . you've watched my kids succeed in ways I never thought they would. Your hard work, patience, and dedication to my children will never go unnoticed or unappreciated. We love you.

To our Framily—you know who you are—thank you for keeping us sane, and not ditching us when we were lost and sometimes crazy. And for only being a phone call away, even when we don't see each other nearly enough. Friends are the family we choose, and I am so glad we chose all of you.

To our families. Dad, thank you for reminding me about the fun side of parenting, which I often forget—and for having the patience I usually don't. Mom, thank you for giving me your determination. I am proud to say I come from a long line of strong women who get things done. Thank you for encouraging that, even when I didn't think I could be. Debbie, thank you for your love and support, and being my second mom, and always being that quick phone call away when things get messy.

Most of all, thank you to my wife, Ashley, for supporting this idea of sharing our story. This has not been an easy journey. Seeing our story written down reminds me that we can get through almost anything—and that we were made to get through this life together, with all of its ups and downs. I cannot do this crazy life with anyone else but you. I love you.

ABOUT THE AUTHOR

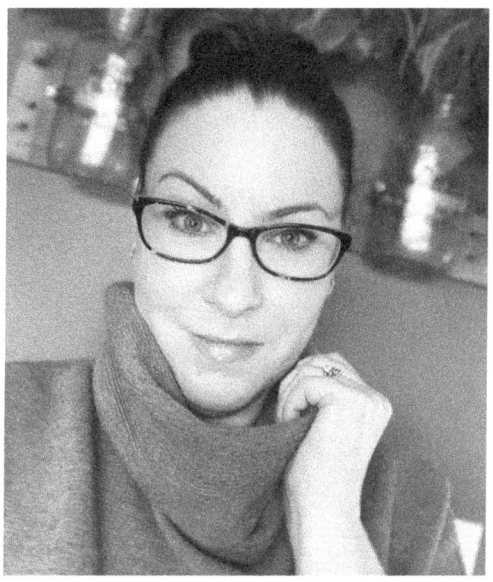

Ashley Biddiscombe is an author and fine artist. She was inspired to write this, her first book, by her personal experiences with infertility, adoption, and parenting children with special needs, hoping to bring awareness to the many private struggles people endure in going through the same.

Interested in getting in touch? You can reach her at @ashleybiddiscombefineart on both Facebook and Instagram, or at her website, www.ashleybiddiscombe.com

CPSIA information can be obtained
at www.ICGtesting.com
Printed in the USA
BVHW040713191022
649666BV00002B/14